From the publishers of the *Tarascon Pocket Pharmacopoeia*®

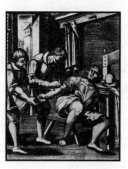

Joseph S. Esherick, MD, FAAFP

Associate Director of Medicine
Medical ICU Director
Ventura County Medical Center
Clinical Associate Professor of Family Medicine
David Geffen School of Medicine
University of California at Los Angeles
California

JONES & BARTLETT
LEARNING

World Headquarters
Jones & Bartlett Learning
40 Tall Pine Drive
Sudbury, MA 01776
978-443-5000
info@jblearning.com
www.jblearning.com

Jones & Bartlett Learning
Canada
6339 Ormindale Way
Mississauga, Ontario L5V 1J2
Canada

Jones & Bartlett Learning
International
Barb House, Barb Mews
London W6 7PA
United Kingdom

Jones & Bartlett Learning books and products are available through most bookstores and online booksellers.
To contact Jones & Bartlett Learning directly, call 800-832-0034, fax 978-443-8000, or visit our website,
www.jblearning.com.

Substantial discounts on bulk quantities of Jones & Bartlett Learning publications are available to
corporations, professional associations, and other qualified organizations. For details and specific
discount information, contact the special sales department at Jones & Bartlett Learning via the above
contact information or send an email to specialsales@jblearning.com.

Library of Congress Cataloging-in-Publication Data

Esherick, Joseph S.
 Tarascon medical procedures pocketbook / by Joseph S. Esherick.
  p. ; cm.
 Medical procedures pocketbook
 Includes bibliographical references and index.
 ISBN-13: 978-1-4496-2648-8
 ISBN-10: 1-4496-2648-3
 1. Clinical medicine—Handbooks, manuals, etc. I. Title. II. Title:
Medical procedures pocketbook.
 [DNLM: 1. Diagnostic Techniques and Procedures—Handbooks. 2. Surgical
Procedures, Operative—Handbooks. WB 39]
 RC55.E84 2012
 616.07'5—dc23

                                          2011013916

6048
Printed in the United States of America
16 15 14 13 12   10 9 8 7 6 5 4 3 2

Production Credits
Executive Publisher: Nancy Anastasi Duffy
Associate Editor: Laura Burns
Senior Production Editor: Daniel Stone
Associate Production Editor: Jill Morton
Marketing Manager: Rebecca Rockel
V.P., Manufacturing and Inventory Control: Therese Connell
Composition: Cenveo Publisher Services
Cover Design: Kate Ternullo
Cover Image: Courtesy of National Library of Medicine
Printing and Binding: Cenveo
Cover Printing: Cenveo

Illustrator
Stephanie Baum

Tarascon Medical Procedures Pocketbook

Contents

	Preface	xiii
	Dedication	xiv
	Reviewers	xv
SECTION I	**PROCEDURAL SEDATION**	**2**
1	**Procedural Sedation**	**3**
	Indications for Procedural Sedation	3
	Contraindications to Procedural Sedation	3
	Airway Assessment for Potentially Difficult Oral Intubation	3
	Procedural Sedation Protocol	5
	Equipment	5
	Anxiolysis in Adults	5
	Options for Moderate–Deep Sedation in Adults	8
	Anxiolysis in Children	8
	Complications	8
	Coding	8
	References	9
SECTION II	**AIRWAY PROCEDURES**	**10**
2	**Endotracheal Intubation**	**11**
	Indications for Intubation	11
	Conditions with Special Considerations for Intubation	11
	Airway Assessment	11
	Predictors of a Difficult Airway	11
	Preparation for Intubation	12
	Equipment	12
	The Seven Ps of Rapid Sequence Intubation	13
	Common Induction Agents	16
	Common Paralytic Agents	16
	Complications	18
	Coding	18
	References	18
3	**Noninvasive Positive-Pressure Ventilation**	**19**
	Definite Indications	19
	Possible Indications	19
	Benefits	19
	Contraindications	19
	Equipment	20
	Modes of Noninvasive Positive-Pressure Ventilation (NPPV)	20
	Technique for BiPAP	20
	Technique for CPAP	22

		Monitoring Patients on NPPV	22
		Predictors of Failure for NPPV	22
		Complications of NPPV	22
		Coding	23
		References	23

SECTION III   CARDIAC PROCEDURES   **24**

4   Pericardiocentesis   **25**
    Etiologies of Pericarditis Associated
      with Large Pericardial Effusions   25
    Indications   25
    Contraindications   25
    Complications   25
    Equipment   26
    Technique   26
    Work-up of Pericarditis   30
    Coding   30
    References   30

5   Synchronized Cardioversion   **31**
    Indications   31
    Contraindications to Elective Cardioversion   31
    Equipment   31
    Technique   32
    Complications   34
    Coding   34
    References   34

6   Transcutaneous Pacing   **35**
    Indications   35
    Contraindications   35
    Equipment   35
    Technique   35
    Complications   37
    Coding   37
    References   37

SECTION IV   DERMATOLOGY PROCEDURES   **38**

7   Laceration Repair   **39**
    Indications   39
    Contraindications   39
    Equipment   39
    Technique   40
    Postprocedure care   44
    Complications   44
    Coding   45
    References   45

8   Cryosurgery of Skin Lesions   **46**
    Indications   46
    Contraindications   46
    Equipment   46
    Technique for Liquid Nitrogen Spray Gun or Cryoprobe   46
    Technique for Q-tip Application   47
    Postprocedure Care   48

	Complications	48
	Coding	48
	References	49
9	**Shave Skin Biopsy**	**50**
	Indications	50
	Contraindications	50
	Equipment	50
	Technique	50
	Postprocedure Care	52
	Complications	52
	Coding	52
	References	52
10	**Excisional Skin Biopsy**	**53**
	Indications	53
	Contraindications	53
	Equipment	53
	Technique	53
	Postprocedure Care	58
	Complications	58
	Coding	58
	References	58
11	**Punch Skin Biopsy**	**59**
	Indications	59
	Contraindications	59
	Complications	59
	Equipment	59
	Technique	60
	Coding	60
	References	62
12	**Ingrown Toenails Removal**	**63**
	Indications	63
	Contraindications	63
	Equipment	63
	Technique	64
	Postprocedure Care	67
	Complications	67
	Coding	68
	References	68
13	**Incision and Drainage of Abscesses**	**69**
	Indications	69
	Contraindications	69
	Equipment	69
	Technique	69
	Complications	72
	Coding	72
	References	72
14	**Lipoma or Subcutaneous Mass Excision**	**73**
	Indications	73
	Contraindications	73
	Complications	73
	Equipment	73
	Enucleation Technique for Small Lipomas	74

	Excision Technique for Large Lipomas or Subcutaneous Masses	75
	Coding	77
	References	77
SECTION V	**EAR, NOSE, AND THROAT PROCEDURES**	**78**
15	**Tympanometry**	**79**
	Indications	79
	Contraindications	79
	Complications	79
	Equipment	79
	Technique	79
	Coding	79
	References	80
16	**Intranasal Device Placement for Epistaxis**	**81**
	Indications	81
	Contraindications	81
	Equipment	81
	Technique	82
	Complications	84
	Coding	85
	References	85
SECTION VI	**GASTROINTESTINAL PROCEDURES**	**86**
17	**Paracentesis**	**87**
	Indications	87
	Contraindications	87
	Equipment	87
	Technique	88
	When to Use Albumin	89
	Ascitic Fluid Analysis	91
	Complications	91
	Coding	92
	References	93
SECTION VII	**GENITOURINARY PROCEDURES**	**94**
18	**No-Scalpel Vasectomy**	**95**
	Indications	95
	Contraindications	95
	Equipment	95
	Technique	95
	Postprocedure Care	100
	Complications	100
	Coding	100
	References	100
19	**Newborn Circumcision with Gomco Clamp**	**101**
	Indications	101
	Contraindications	101
	Equipment	101
	Technique	102
	Postprocedure Care	105

Contents   ix

	Complications	106
	Coding	106
	References	107

SECTION VIII **GYNECOLOGIC PROCEDURES**   **108**

20 **Pap Smear**   **109**
	Indications	109
	Relative Contraindications	109
	Equipment	109
	Technique of Traditional Pap Smear	109
	Technique of Liquid-based Pap Smear	112
	Postprocedure Evaluation	113
	Complications	113
	Coding	113
	References	113

21 **Endometrial Biopsy**   **114**
	Indications	114
	Contraindications	114
	Equipment	114
	Technique	114
	Postprocedure Care	117
	Complications	117
	Coding	117
	References	117

22 **Intrauterine Device Insertion and Removal**   **118**
	Intrauterine Device Insertion	
	Indications	118
	Contraindications	118
	Equipment	118
	Technique	119
	Postprocedure Care	121
	Complications	124
	Coding	124
	Intrauterine Device Removal	
	Indications	124
	Contraindications	124
	Equipment	124
	Technique	124
	Postprocedure Care	125
	Complications	125
	Coding	125
	References	125

SECTION IX **HEMATOLOGY/ONCOLOGY PROCEDURES**   **126**

23 **Bone Marrow Aspiration and Biopsy**   **127**
	Indications	127
	Contraindications	127
	Equipment	127
	Biopsy Sites	128
	Technique for Posterior Superior Iliac Spine Bone Marrow Aspirate	129

                    Technique for Posterior Superior Iliac
                        Spine Bone Marrow Core Biopsy   130
                    Bone Marrow Aspirate Optional Studies   133
                    Complications   133
                    Coding   133
                    References   133

SECTION X   NEUROLOGY PROCEDURES   134

        24   Lumbar Puncture   135
                Indications   135
                Contraindications   135
                Equipment   135
                Technique   136
                Cerebrospinal Fluid Studies   138
                When to Obtain a CT Scan of the Head Prior to a
                    Lumbar Puncture   138
                Predictors of Bacterial Meningitis   139
                Complications   139
                Coding   139
                References   139

SECTION XI   ORTHOPEDICS PROCEDURES   140

        25   Splinting and Casting of the Extremities   141
                Indications for Splinting   141
                Indications for Casting   141
                Contraindications   141
                Equipment   141
                Basic Technique for Splinting Extremities   142
                Basic Technique for Casting Extremities   144
                Postprocedure Care   151
                Complications   151
                Coding   151
                References   152

        26   Arthrocentesis   153
                Indications for Diagnostic Arthrocentesis   153
                Indications for Therapeutic Arthrocentesis   153
                Absolute Contraindications   153
                Relative Contraindications   153
                Equipment   153
                Technique for Knee Arthrocentesis   154
                Technique for Shoulder Arthrocentesis   155
                Technique for Elbow Arthrocentesis   156
                Synovial Fluid Analysis   158
                Complications   158
                Coding   158
                References   158

        27   Joint Injections   159
                Indications   159
                Contraindications   159
                Equipment   159
                General Technique for All Injections   159
                Technique of Glenohumeral Joint Injection   160
                Technique of Knee Injection   160

Contents

	Technique of Subacromial Bursa Injection	160
	Technique for Lateral Epicondyle Injection	162
	Technique for Trochanteric Bursa Injection	163
	Post-Procedure Care	163
	Complications	163
	Coding	163
	References	163
SECTION XII	**PULMONARY PROCEDURES**	**164**
28	**Spirometry**	**165**
	Indications	165
	Contraindications	165
	Equipment	165
	Technique	165
	Acceptability Criteria	166
	Reproducibility Criteria	166
	Interpretation of Results	167
	Complications	168
	Coding	168
	References	168
29	**Thoracentesis**	**169**
	Indications	169
	Contraindications	169
	Equipment	169
	Technique	170
	Pleural Fluid Analysis (Table 29-1)	173
	Complications	173
	Coding	174
	References	174
30	**Basics of Mechanical Ventilation**	**175**
	Initiating Mechanical Ventilation	175
	General Guidelines for Mechanical Ventilation	176
	Complications of Mechanical Ventilation	176
	Coding	178
	References	178
31	**Tube Thoracostomy**	**179**
	Indications	179
	Contraindications	179
	Equipment	179
	Technique	180
	Chest Tube Troubleshooting	182
	Discontinuation of Chest Tubes	184
	Complications of Tube Thoracostomy	185
	Coding	185
	References	185
SECTION XIII	**VASCULAR PROCEDURES**	**186**
32	**Central Venous Access**	**187**
	Indications for Central Venous Catheters	187
	Contraindications of Central Venous Catheter Placement	187
	Equipment	187
	General Technique for Central Line Placement in All Locations	188

Internal Jugular Vein Catheters	192
Subclavian Vein Catheters	193
Femoral Vein Catheters	194
Complications	195
Coding	196
References	196

33 Arterial Line Placement   197
Indications	197
Contraindications	197
Equipment	197
Technique for Radial Arterial Line	198
Technique for Femoral or Brachial Arterial Lines	199
Complications	202
Coding	202
References	202

34 Pulmonary Artery Catheter Insertion   203
Indications	203
Absolute Contraindications	203
Relative Contraindications	203
Equipment	203
Technique	204
Complications	208
Coding	208
References	208

35 Intraosseous Line Placement   209
Indications	209
Contraindications	209
Equipment	209
Technique	210
Complications	212
Coding	212
References	212

Index   213

■ PREFACE

The *Tarascon Medical Procedures Pocketbook* is an evidence-based, point-of-care guide to the most commonly performed ambulatory care and hospital procedures. This pocket reference provides busy clinicians and students a resource for the indications, contraindications, necessary equipment, step-by-step technique, fluid analysis, complications, and coding for the most commonly performed medical procedures. This pocketbook is packed with over 200 tables and figures that depict the proper technique used for performing each procedure.

The *Tarascon Medical Procedures Pocketbook* is the only comprehensive reference book for medical procedures that fits in your shirt pocket. As such, it is an essential portable guide for all clinicians, medical students, residents, and midlevel providers who perform medical procedures in either the outpatient or inpatient setting.

I would like to thank my editorial board, without whom this project would not have been possible. Their countless clinical pearls have been incorporated into this pocketbook. I would also like to thank the hospital librarian, Janet Parker, who has acquired virtually every reference article that was used for the preparation of this manuscript.

The information within this pocketbook has been compiled from sources believed to be reliable. Nevertheless, the *Tarascon Medical Procedures Pocketbook* is intended to be a clinical guide only; it is not meant to be a replacement for sound clinical judgment. Although painstaking efforts have been made to find all errors and omissions, some errors may remain. If you find an error or wish to make a suggestion, please email your comments to editor@tarascon.com.

Best wishes,

Joseph S. Esherick, MD, FAAFP

■ DEDICATION

I would like to dedicate this book to all of the current and former residents of the Ventura Family Medicine Residency Program, who continually inspire me to strive for excellence.

■ REVIEWERS

Tarascon Medical Procedures Pocketbook

SECTION I	PROCEDURAL SEDATION	2
SECTION II	AIRWAY PROCEDURES	10
SECTION III	CARDIAC PROCEDURES	24
SECTION IV	DERMATOLOGY PROCEDURES	38
SECTION V	EAR, NOES, AND THROAT PROCEDURES	78
SECTION VI	GASTROINTESTINAL PROCEDURES	86
SECTION VII	GENITOURINARY PROCEDURES	94
SECTION VIII	GYNECOLOGIC PROCEDURES	108
SECTION IX	HEMATOLOGY/ONCOLOGY PROCEDURES	126
SECTION X	NEUROLOGY PROCEDURES	134
SECTION XI	ORTHOPEDICS PROCEDURES	140
SECTION XII	PULMONARY PROCEDURES	164
SECTION XIII	VASCULAR PROCEDURES	186

SECTION I

PROCEDURAL SEDATION

1 ■ PROCEDURAL SEDATION

INDICATIONS FOR PROCEDURAL SEDATION

- Patient factors: Anxiety, preexisting pain
- Procedure factors: Painful, requires motionless patient, duration
- Common inpatient procedures that may require procedural sedation
  - Nonemergent chest tube placement
  - Bone marrow biopsy and aspiration
  - Synchronized dc cardioversion
  - Biopsy or incision and drainage procedures
  - Deep line placement
  - Laceration repair
  - Extensive burn debridement
  - Foreign body removal
  - Shoulder, elbow, or hip dislocations
  - Fracture reductions
  - CT or MRI scan sedation
  - Any procedure that **MAY** cause pain or anxiety

CONTRAINDICATIONS TO PROCEDURAL SEDATION

- Patient refuses or is incapable of providing informed consent
- Hemodynamic instability
- Respiratory distress

AIRWAY ASSESSMENT FOR POTENTIALLY DIFFICULT ORAL INTUBATION

- Establish the airway Mallampati Class (**Figure 1-1**).
- Neck extension ≥ 70° (patient should be able to see ceiling above his or her body)
- 3-3-2 rule
  - Jaw opening: Can fit three fingers between teeth with mouth wide open
  - Chin length: Chin should be at least three finger-widths long
  - Thyromental distance: Should be at least two finger-widths long
- Potentially difficult airway if: Mallampati Class III–IV, poor neck extension/jaw opening, short chin/thyromental distance, macroglossia, oral or neck mass, dysmorphic facial features, high-arched palate, short neck, neck circumference > 17 inches, and a history of obstructive sleep apnea or difficult intubations

TABLE 1-1. Levels of Sedation

Sedation Score	Sedation Level	Level of consciousness	Response to verbal	Response to tactile	Airway patency	Ventilation and oxygenation
0	None	Fully aware	P	P	P	P
1	Light	Sedated	P–L	P	P	P
2	Moderate	Somnolent	L–A	P–L	P–L*	P–L*
3	Deep	Obtunded	A	L (noxious)	L–A	L
4	General anesthesia	Unconscious	A	A	A	L–A

P = Present/Normal; L = Limited/mildly abnormal; A = Absent/inadequate

* = May need supplemental oxygen

Source: Data from American Society of Anesthesiologists. Continuum of Depth of Sedation: Definition of General Anesthesia and Levels of Sedation/Analgesia. Standards Guidelines and Statements. http://www.asahq.org/publicationsAndServices/sgstoc.htm. Accessed January 28, 2011.

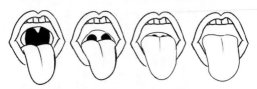

FIGURE 1-1. Airway Assessment for Potentially Difficult Oral Intubation
Adapted from Mallampati SR, Gatt SP, Gugino LD, et al. A Clinical Sign to Predict Difficulty Tracheal Intubation: A Prospective Study. *Can J Anaesth.* 1985; 32(4): 430, Figure 1.

- Mallampati Class: Have patient open mouth while sitting, stick out tongue, and say "ah."
- Visualize lowest anatomic structure: Mnemonic is PUSH.
  - Anterior Tonsillar Pillars (Class I); Uvula (Class II); Soft palate (Class III); Hard palate (Class IV)

PROCEDURAL SEDATION PROTOCOL

- Check a pregnancy test on women of childbearing age.
- No clear liquids for ≥ 2 hours or food for ≥ 6 hours.
- Monitor continuous heart rate and oximetry.
- Monitor blood pressure and level of consciousness every 5–10 minutes.

EQUIPMENT

- Suction equipment
- Supplemental oxygen
- Oral airway and nasal trumpet
- Bag-valve mask, emergency airway cart, crash cart
- Pulse oximeter
- Cardiac and blood pressure monitors
- End-tidal CO_2 monitor (if available)

ANXIOLYSIS IN ADULTS (SEE TABLE 1-1 AND TABLE 1-2)

- Midazolam or lorazepam

TABLE 1-2. Medications for Procedural Sedation in Adults

Drug	Bolus IV Dosing	Titration IV Dosing	Benefits	Side Effects	Contraindications
Morphine	2–4 mg	2 mg q 3–5 min	• Analgesia • Sedation	• Hypotension • Itching	• Both opiates and benzodiazepines
Fentanyl	0.5–1 mcg/kg (≤ 100 mcg)	0.25–0.5 mcg/kg (≤ 50 mcg) q 3–5 min		• Fentanyl: chest wall rigidity	• Hypotension • Obtundation • Respiratory depression
Midazolam	2–4 mg	1–2 mg q 5 min	• Anxiolysis • Amnesia	• Hypotension • Paradoxical disinhibition	
Lorazepam	2–4 mg	1–2 mg q 5 min			
Ketamine	1–1.5 mg/kg IV bolus over 1–2 min; may give additional 0.5 mg/kg IV if needed IV Premedication: • Midazolam 1–2 mg IV (↓ emergence reactions) • Glycopyrrolate 0.1 mg IV (↓ salivation)		• Amnesia • Analgesia • Anxiolysis • No resp. depression • Broncho-dilates	• Emergence reactions (8%) • Hypersalivation • Tachycardia • Hypertension • Increased ICP • Increased IOP	• Tracheal/laryngeal disease • Respiratory tract infection • CAD/CHF/marked HTN • Potentially increased ICP • Glaucoma or globe injury • Psychosis • Seizure or thyroid disorder • Porphyria

Propofol	1 mg/kg bolus then 0.5 mg/kg q 2–3 min prn • Caution in children < 12 years	• Broncho-dilates • ↓ ICP	• Hypotension (7%) • Apnea (3–4%) • Injection pain	• Allergy to eggs or soy products
"Ketofol" (ketamine + propofol)	1:1 mixture of ketamine (10 mg/ml) and propofol (10 mg/ml); 2–3 ml IV q 30–60 seconds titrated to effect; usually requires about 0.75 mg/kg of each medication	• As above • Less ↓ BP • Less apnea	• Emergence reactions • Hypersalivation • ↑ HR/BP/ICP/IOP	• See above for individual medication components
Etomidate	0.1 mg/kg	0.05 mg/kg q 3–5 min × 2 (max dose: 0.2 mg/kg) • ↓ ICP	• Vomiting • Myoclonus (20%) • Adrenal suppression	• Adrenal insufficiency • Known hypersensitivity • Age < 10 years (relative)

HR = heart rate, BP = blood pressure, ICP = intracranial pressure, IOP = intraocular pressure, HTN = hypertension

• Give opiates at full dose, then titrate benzodiazepines after administration of opiates
• Antidote for opiate overdose: naloxone 0.01 mg/kg IV
• Antidote for benzodiazepine overdose: flumazenil 0.01 mg/kg (max 1 mg) IV; avoid if chronic benzodiazepine use or seizure disorder

Source: Information from *Ann Emer Med.* 2004; 44: 460–471, and *Ann Emer Med.* 2005; 45: 177–196, and *Ann Emer Med.* 2007; 49: 15–36.

OPTIONS FOR MODERATE–DEEP SEDATION IN ADULTS (SEE TABLE 1-1 AND TABLE 1-2)

- Opiates (fentanyl or morphine) **AND** benzodiazepines (midazolam or lorazepam)
- Ketamine and midazolam
- Ketamine and propofol (Ketofol)
- Propofol +/− fentanyl
- Etomidate +/− fentanyl

ANXIOLYSIS IN CHILDREN (SEE TABLE 1-1 AND TABLE 1-2)

- Midazolam
  - Oral: 0.5 mg/kg (max. 15 mg) of IV formulation; more palatable if served cold and mixed with acetaminophen elixir 15 mg/kg
  - Intranasal: 0.4 mg/kg (max. 12 mg)
  - IV: 0.025–0.05 mg/kg q 3–5 minutes (max. 0.4 mg/kg)
  - Rectal suppository: 0.25–0.5 mg/kg (max. 15 mg)
- Chloral hydrate for diagnostic imaging procedures in children < 3 years
  - 50–75 mg/kg PO and additional 25–50 mg/kg if needed after 30 minutes
  - Not to exceed 2 gm or 100 mg/kg PO

COMPLICATIONS

- Respiratory depression
- Hypotension
- Nausea/vomiting (usually opioid-related)
- Parodoxical disinhibition from benzodiazepines

CODING

99144	Moderate procedural sedation provided by same physician performing diagnostic or therapeutic service—first 30 minutes
99145	Each additional 15 minutes
99147	Moderate procedural sedation provided by a physician other than the physician performing diagnostic or therapeutic service—first 30 minutes
99150	Each additional 15 minutes

REFERENCES

NEJM. 2000; 342: 938–945.
Ann Emer Med. 2004; 44: 460–471.
Ann Emer Med. 2005; 45: 177–196.
Pediatrics. 2002; 109: 894–897.
Ann Emer Med. 2007; 49: 15–36.
Emerg Med Clin N Amer. 2005; 23: 509–517.
Ann Emer Med. 2007; 49: 454–467.

SECTION II

AIRWAY PROCEDURES

2 ■ ENDOTRACHEAL INTUBATION

INDICATIONS FOR INTUBATION

- Unable to protect airway
- Hypercapneic respiratory failure
- Hypoxic respiratory failure
- Cardiac or respiratory arrest
- Need to maintain hyperventilation
  - Closed head injury
  - Severe metabolic acidosis

CONDITIONS WITH SPECIAL CONSIDERATIONS FOR INTUBATION

- Inability to extend neck
  - Known or suspected C-spine or basilar skull fracture (cervical immobilization) or a fused neck: Consider fiberoptic oral intubation or video laryngoscopy.
- Uncontrolled oropharyngeal hemorrhage or tracheal or laryngeal fracture
  - Often requires a surgical airway
- Mandibular fracture, trismus, or limited jaw opening
  - May require fiberoptic oral intubation or nasotracheal intubation

AIRWAY ASSESSMENT

- Determine the patient's Mallampati airway class (see **Figure 1-1**, page **05**).
- Assess neck extension ($\geq 70°$ is normal).
- 3-3-2 rule
  - Jaw opening: Three finger-widths between teeth with mouth wide open
  - Chin length: At least three finger-widths
  - Thyromental distance: At least two finger-widths

PREDICTORS OF A DIFFICULT AIRWAY

- **History**
  - Stridor
  - Active oral or airway bleeding
  - Obstructive sleep apnea
  - Rheumatoid arthritis or ankylosing spondylitis with cervical spine involvement
  - Dysmorphic facial features

- Down Syndrome
- Head and neck tumor
- Prior neck surgery or radiation therapy
- History of prior difficult intubations, tracheal stenosis, or tracheostomy
- **Exam Features**
  - High arched palate
  - Low-set ears
  - Thick jowls or short neck
  - Marked facial distortion
  - Macroglossia
  - Small mandible
  - Limited ability to open mouth
  - Mallampati Class III–IV: poor neck extension, narrow jaw opening, short thryomental length

PREPARATION FOR INTUBATION

- Confirm code status of patient.
- Explain procedure to patient if semielective intubation.
- Confirm a functional IV line.
- Check equipment including laryngoscope, suction, and endotracheal tube cuff.
- Place patient on monitor with cardiac rhythm and continuous oximetry.
- Place patient supine with head at top of bed.
- Remove dentures.

EQUIPMENT

- Cardiac monitor, pulse oximeter, and blood pressure monitoring
- Gloves
- Mask and protective eyeware
- Suction system connected to a Yankauer suction tip
- Bag-valve mask connected to oxygen source
- Oral airway
- Water-soluble lubricant (for endotracheal tube tip)
- Endotracheal tube with stylet
  - Tube size in children = (age in years + 4)/4 or size equal to pinky fingernail.
  - Use uncuffed tube for tube size < 5.5 mm or for children under 8 years old.
  - Adult men size 7.5–8; adult women size 7–7.5.
- 10-ml syringe
- End-tidal CO_2 detector
- Endotracheal tube-securing device (strap or tape)
- Stethoscope

- Laryngoscope with Macintosh blades (sizes 3 and 4) and Miller blades (sizes 2 and 3)
- Frova or Eschmann stylet available as intubating adjuncts
- Intermediate airway available (e.g., appropriate sizes of laryngeal mask airways)

THE SEVEN PS OF RAPID SEQUENCE INTUBATION

- Preparation (IV access, medications, equipment, monitor, patient position)
  - If no cervical spine injury, put patient into the "sniffing position" (flexed neck and extended head) (**Figure 2-1**).
  - Raise bed so that the mouth is at the level of your xiphoid notch.
  - If BMI > 30, consider placing patient in a "ramped" position, which lowers the pannus and can improve visualization (**Figure 2-2**).
- Preoxygenation with 100% oxygen (three minutes if possible)
- Pretreatment (LOAD mnemonic)
  - Lidocaine 1.5 mg/kg IVP two–three min before intubation (if suspected increased intracranial pressure or reactive airway disease)
  - Opiates (fentanyl 2–3 mcg/kg slow IVP over one–two min for significant CAD, hypertensive emergencies, or aortic dissections)
  - Atropine (0.02 mg/kg atropine [minimum, 0.1 mg; maximum, 0.5 mg] IV for children ≤ 10 years)
  - Defasciculating agent (e.g., rocuronium or vecuronium 1 mg IVP) a consideration if increased intracranial pressure
- Protection (from aspiration) with cricoid pressure (Sellick maneuver)
- Paralysis with a neuromuscular blocking agent after an induction agent given
- Placement of tube (45–60 seconds after paralytic)
  - Open mouth and introduce laryngoscope blade using left hand to proper position (**Figure 2-3**).
- Proof: end-tidal CO_2 detector and chest x-ray confirmation of tube placement
    - Introduce Macintosh blade in the right side of the mouth; sweep tongue to the left; place tip in the vallecula.
    - Introduce Miller blade in the center of the mouth; place tip under the epiglottis.
  - Elevate the laryngoscope blade upward and forward to visualize the vocal cords.
    - If cords are not visualized, can try the following: pull back laryngoscope blade and larynx may fall into view; put patient into a better "sniffing position;" have an assistant perform a BURP maneuver (tracheal cartilage pushed Backward, Upward, and Rightward, and then Pressure applied); or change laryngoscope blade.
  - Intubate without bagging if possible (**Figure 2-4**).

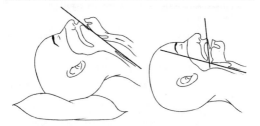

FIGURE 2-1. Proper Sniffing Position for Endotracheal Intubation
Adapted from Kabrhel C, Thomsen TW, Setnik GS, et al. Orotracheal Intubation. *N Engl J Med.* 2007; 356(17): e16, Figure 2.

A. Poor alignment of the oropharyngeal and laryngeal axes with head in neutral position
B. A towel or pillow under the occiput, raising the head about 4 inches off the bed, provides good alignment of the oropharyngeal and laryngeal axes with the head in a sniffing position (neck flexed and head extended)

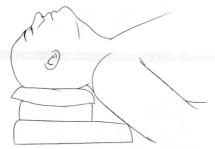

FIGURE 2-2. "Ramp" Position for Intubation in Morbidly Obese Patients
Adapted from Rich JM. Use of an Elevation Pillow to Produce the Head-Elevated Laryngoscopy Position for Airway Management in Morbidly Obese and Large-Framed Patients. *Anaesth Anal.* 2004; 98(1): 265, Figure 1.

A standard intubation pillow in conjunction with elevation pillow. Elevation of the shoulders and upper back facilitates alignment of the laryngeal, pharyngeal and oral axis of the airway in morbidly obese and large framed patients.

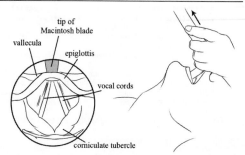

FIGURE 2-3. Introduction of a Macintosh Blade for Direct Laryngoscopy

A Macintosh laryngoscope blade is introduced along the right side of the mouth. The blade is then brought toward the center to sweep the tongue to the left as it is gradually advanced toward the larynx. The tip of the Macintosh blade is placed in the vallecula and then the laryngoscope is lifted up and forward to expose the glottis. The inset identifies the most important glottic structures.

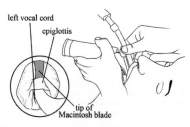

FIGURE 2-4. Insertion of an Endotracheal Tube

An endotracheal tube is inserted along the right side of the mouth while directly visualizing the glottis and vocal cords. Passage along the right side of the mouth prevents obscuring the direct visualization of the glottis. A stylet is typically inserted into the endotracheal tube to increase its rigidity. The inset shows the tube passing through the vocal cords.

- • If only the corniculate tubercles are seen, an Eschmann or Frova
    stylet can be placed anterior to the tubercles and used as a stylet
    to introduce the endotracheal tube.
  - • Abort intubation and bag mask ventilate patient if SaO_2 falls
    below 90% during attempt.
  - • Depth of insertion is 3–4 cm beyond cords; usually 22 cm +/– 2
    cm in adults.
  - • Inflate the endotracheal tube cuff with 10 ml air (**Figure 2-5**) and
    secure tube in place with tape or a specialized strap (**Figure 2-6**).
  - • Listen for equal breath sounds and listen over stomach; assure good
    chest rise; and confirm color change on an end-tidal CO_2 detector
    (purple to yellow).
- • Post-intubation management (ongoing sedation and check chest x-ray)

COMMON INDUCTION AGENTS

- • Etomidate
  - • Dose: 0.2–0.3 mg/kg IVP over 30 seconds (20 mg in adults)
  - • Benefits: no hemodynamic effects, decreases intracranial pressure
    (ICP)
  - • Drawbacks: can cause vomiting, myoclonus, and transient adrenal
    suppression
- • Propofol
  - • Dose: 1–2 mg/kg IV (2.5 mg/kg IV if no paralytics used)
  - • Benefits: decreases ICP, bronchodilates, antiemetic, and anticonvulsant
  - • Drawbacks: hypotension (prehydrate patient), myoclonus, and tremors
- • Midazolam
  - • Dosing: 0.2–0.3 mg/kg (up to 10 mg) IV bolus
  - • Benefits: rapid onset and may offer cerebroprotection during intubation
  - • Drawbacks: negative inotrope, potential for hypotension, and fre-
    quently underdosed
- • Ketamine
  - • Dosing: 1.5 mg/kg IV bolus over one–two minutes
  - • Benefits: no respiratory depression, maintains airway patency,
    bronchodilates
  - • Drawbacks: increases intracranial and intraocular pressure, blood
    pressure, and heart rate; hypersalivation; emergence reactions
  - • Premedication: midazolam 2 mg IVP and glycopyrrolate 0.1 mg IVP or
    atropine 0.1 mg/kg (max 0.5 mg) IVP

COMMON PARALYTIC AGENTS

- • Succinylcholine (depolarizing neuromuscular blocker)
  - • Dosing: 1.5 mg/kg IVP
  - • Benefits: rapid-acting and short duration

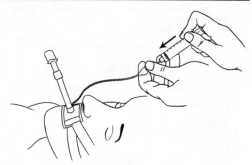

FIGURE 2-5. Inflating Endotracheal Tube Cuff

A 10-ml syringe is used to inflate the endotracheal tube cuff. The bulb should be firm after inflating the endotracheal tube cuff.

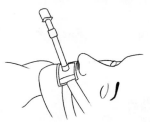

FIGURE 2-6. Securing Endotracheal Tube

The endotracheal tube is secured in place with a strap.

- Drawbacks: increases ICP and intraocular pressure (blunted with lidocaine), malignant hyperthermia, prolonged paralysis if pseudo-cholinesterase deficiency
- Avoid with hyperkalemia, congenital myopathies, neuromuscular disorders, or 24 hours after severe burns, crush injuries, or spinal cord injuries

- Rocuronium (nondepolarizing neuromuscular blocker if succinylcholine contraindicated)
  - Dosing: 0.6–1 mg/kg IVP; duration is 20–75 minutes
  - Benefits: shortest-acting of the nondepolarizing neuromuscular blockers
  - Drawbacks: duration of action is at least 20 minutes long

COMPLICATIONS

- Hypotension: risk factors include sepsis, COPD, and low body weight
- Hypertension
- Bradycardia
- Cardiac arrest
- Cardiac arrhythmias
- Esophageal intubation
- Laryngospasm
- Vocal cord trauma or vocal cord dysfunction
- Oral trauma: injury to teeth, lips, or larynx
- Tracheal or esophageal perforation (by stylet)
- Aspiration pneumonitis
- Cervical spine injury (with excessive neck manipulation in trauma patients)
- Pneumothorax (from aggressive bag-valve mask ventilation in patients with poor lung compliance)
- Sinusitis

CODING

31500   Intubation

REFERENCES

Anesthesiol. 2004; 101: 565.
Anaesthesia. 2004; 59: 675.
Acad Emer Med. 2003; 10: 329.
NEJM. 2007; 356: e15.
Chest. 2005; 127: 1397.
Amer J Emer Med. 2008; 26: 845.
Lancet. 2009; 374: 293.
Crit Care Med. 2006; 34: 2355.
Anesth Analg. 2004; 98: 264.
Emer Clin N Amer. 2008; 26: 1043.
Emerg Med J. 2005; 22: 815–816.

3 ■ NONINVASIVE POSITIVE-PRESSURE VENTILATION

DEFINITE INDICATIONS (LEVEL 1 EVIDENCE)

- Severe CHF exacerbations
- Moderate—severe COPD exacerbations

POSSIBLE INDICATIONS (LEVEL 2 EVIDENCE)

- Acute hypoxemic respiratory failure (not Acute Respiratory Distress Syndrome)
- CHF or COPD exacerbations with a Do-Not-Intubate code status
- Acute respiratory failure in immunocompromised patients (AIDS or chronic immunosuppression)
- Facilitation of ventilator-weaning in patients intubated for a COPD exacerbation

BENEFITS

- Reduces mortality (especially in CHF and COPD exacerbations)
- Decreases the incidence of nosocomial infections
- Lowers the frequency of invasive mechanical ventilation

CONTRAINDICATIONS

- Cardiac or respiratory arrest
- Inability to protect airway
- Copious respiratory secretions
- Upper airway obstruction
- Uncooperative/agitated patients
- Hemodynamic instability or life-threatening arrhythmias
- Severe nausea, vomiting, or increased risk of aspiration
- Recent gastroesophageal, facial, or upper airway surgery
- Significant upper gastrointestinal bleed
- Facial deformities precluding a tight mask application
- Facial burns
- Significant claustrophobia
- Depressed level of consciousness or significant encephalopathy (relative contraindication)
    - Patient must have constant bedside monitoring if noninvasive ventilation is used in this setting.

EQUIPMENT

- BiPAP machine
- Various facial masks
- Airway tubing
- Supplemental oxygen

MODES OF NONINVASIVE POSITIVE-PRESSURE VENTILATION (NPPV)

- **Continuous Positive Airway Pressure (CPAP)**
  - As effective as BiPAP for CHF exacerbations
- **Bilevel Positive Airway Pressure (BiPAP)**
  - Preferred for COPD exacerbations or acute hypoxemic respiratory failure.
  - Adjust iPAP and ePAP levels.
  - Pressure support = iPAP − ePAP.

TECHNIQUE FOR BIPAP

- Machine cycles between a high pressure-level (iPAP) and a low pressure-level (ePAP).
- Use a mask-fitting wheel to determine the optimal mask size for the patient (**Figure 3-1**).

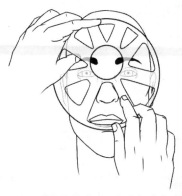

FIGURE 3-1. Using a Mask Fitting Wheel to Determine Optimal Face Mask Size

- Machine Settings
  - iPAP (started typically at 8–10 cm H_2O).
  - ePAP (started typically at 4–5 cm H_2O).
  - Triggering sensitivity is the sensitivity at which the patient triggers iPAP.
  - Rise time is the rate at which air flow occurs during inspiration (range = 0.05–0.4 seconds).
- Critical to prepare patient adequately prior to initiation of BiPAP.
  - Slowly acclimate patients to BiPAP.
  - Start by having patients hold the mask to face.
  - Secure mask in place (**Figure 3-2**).
- Titrate iPAP in increments of 2 cm H_2O to achieve:
  - Tidal volume (Vt) = 5–7 ml/kg predicted body weight (PBW).
    - PBW in kg (♀) = 45.5 + [2.3 × (height in inches − 60)]
    - PBW in kg (♂) = 50 + [2.3 × (height in inches − 60)]
  - Respiratory rate < 25 bpm.
  - Decreased work of breathing and improved vital signs.
  - Aim to keep peak inspiratory pressure (PIP) < 20 cm H_2O.
  - Use caution with iPAP > 20 cm H_2O (especially > 25 cm H_2O) due to increased risk of gastric insufflation.
- Titrate FiO_2 to achieve $SaO_2 \geq 90\%$.
- Increase ePAP to allow weaning of the FiO_2; ideally desire long-term $FiO_2 \leq 0.6$.
- Adjust rise time and triggering sensitivity titrated to patient comfort.

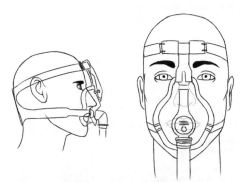

FIGURE 3-2. Bilevel Positive Airway Pressure (BiPAP) Face Mask Strapped In Place

TECHNIQUE FOR CPAP

- Initiate CPAP at 8–10 cm H_2O.
- Titrate FiO_2 to achieve $SaO_2 \geq 90\%$.
- Increase CPAP as tolerated to achieve:
  - Respiratory rate < 25 bpm
  - Decreased work of breathing and improved vital signs

MONITORING PATIENTS ON NPPV

- "Eyeball" test to examine for any of the following:
  - Dyspnea, increased work of breathing or diaphoresis
  - Patient comfort, tolerance of mask or presence of anxiety
  - Any patient-ventilator dyssynchrony
  - Any significant air leaks
- Vital signs and continuous cardiac rhythm monitoring
- Continuous oximetry
- Arterial blood gas (ABG) at baseline, after one–two hours and as indicated
  - The ABG should be significantly improved after 1 hour of NPPV.
  - If the pulmonary status is unimproved after one–two hours, consider endotracheal intubation.

PREDICTORS OF FAILURE FOR NPPV

- Poor patient cooperation
- Patient intolerance of face mask
- Low body mass index ≤ 23
- Edentulous patients or marked facial deformities
- Presence of significant encephalopathy or dementia
- Inability to coordinate breathing with ventilator
- Simplified Acute Physiology Score II (SAPS II) ≥ 35
- APACHE II score > 20–23
- Presence of Acute Respiratory Distress Syndrome (ARDS)
- $PaO_2/FiO_2 < 150$ or minimal improvement in respiratory acidosis after one hour of NPPV

COMPLICATIONS OF NPPV

- **Minor Complications**
  - Nasal or sinus congestion
  - Sinus or ear pain
  - Conjunctival irritation
  - Pressure sores of nasal bridge or facial skin (11%)
  - Gastric insufflation

- **Major Complications (< 5%)**
  - Severe gastric distension (rare if iPAP < 25 cm H_2O)
  - Pulmonary aspiration
  - Pneumothorax
  - Pressure ulcers of face
  - Hypotension

CODING

94005   Ventilator management (applies to titration of noninvasive positive pressure ventilation)

REFERENCES

JAMA. 2005; 294: 3124–3130.
Crit Care Med. 2007; 35: 2402–2407.
Crit Care Med. 2008; 36: 789–794.
Curr Opin. Crit Care. 2007; 13: 12–19.
Ann Emerg Med. 2007; 50: 666–675.
Crit Care Med. 2007; 35: 932–939.

SECTION III

CARDIAC PROCEDURES

4 ■ PERICARDIOCENTESIS

ETIOLOGIES OF PERICARDITIS ASSOCIATED WITH LARGE PERICARDIAL EFFUSIONS

- Common causes of cardiac tamponade in the United States: idiopathic or viral pericarditis; malignancy; rheumatic diseases; and uremia
- Other causes: infectious (tuberculous [cause of up to 14% of cardiac tamponade in developing countries], bacterial, fungal, rickettsial or fungal); Dressler's syndrome; post-irradiation; chest trauma; post-pericardiotomy; hypothyroidism; and meds (hydralazine, isoniazid, methyldopa, phenytoin, and procainamide).

INDICATIONS

- Diagnostic
  - To determine the etiology of an unexplained pericardial effusion
- Therapeutic
  - Relief of cardiac tamponade (a pulsus paradoxus > 12 mm Hg or a ratio of paradoxical pulse/pulse pressure that exceeds 50% are both abnormal)

CONTRAINDICATIONS

- Small asymptomatic pericardial effusion (less than 200 ml)
- Loculated pericardial effusion
- Absence of an anterior pericardial effusion
- Acute traumatic hemopericardium
- Coagulopathy
  - INR > 1.4 or PTT > 1.5 times the upper limit of normal
- Thrombocytopenia (platelet count < 50,000)

COMPLICATIONS

- Cardiac puncture
- Laceration of a coronary artery
- Liver laceration
- Cardiac arrhythmias
- Hemothorax
- Pneumothorax
- Infection
- Air embolus

EQUIPMENT

- Prepackaged pericardiocentesis kit containing: introducer needle, J wire, dilator, catheter guide, 8 Fr drainage catheter, drainage bag, three-way stopcock, 60-ml aspirating syringe, and sterile collection tubes
- Echocardiogram (for echocardiogram-guided pericardiocentesis)
- Sterile prep: chlorhexidine or povidone-iodine swabs
- Sterile drape or towels
- Sterile gown and gloves
- Surgeon's cap and mask
- 1% lidocaine with or without epinephrine, with 10-ml syringe and needles
- Sterile ECG monitoring cord with alligator clip
- Cardiac monitor
- Sterile bandage
- No. 11 scalpel
- 2-0 nylon suture

TECHNIQUE

- Informed consent.
- Perform a "time out" to confirm the correct patient and procedure.
- Place patient supine with the head of bed elevated to 45°.
- Sterile prep and drape of the lower chest and subxiphoid area.
- Anesthetize the insertion site 0.5 cm left of the xiphoid tip with 1% lidocaine.
- Attach one end of the sterile ECG cord to the pericardiocentesis needle using an alligator clip and the other end to the V_1 or V_5 precordial lead using another alligator clip.
- Assure proper functioning of the cardiac monitor.
- Advance the introducer needle connected to a syringe at a 30–45° angle to the skin with constant negative pressure. Aim toward the left shoulder (**Figure 4-1**).
  - Echocardiogram used for real-time ultrasound-guided pericardiocentesis.
  - Typical depth of insertion from the skin to the pericardium is 6–8 cm.
  - Negative deflection of the QRS complex, or ST segment depression, occurs when the needle touches the pericardial sac.
  - Stop advancing the needle when pericardial fluid is obtained.
    - Pericardial fluid does not clot in cases of hemopericardium.
  - ST segment elevation signifies needle contact with the epicardium/myocardium, and the needle should be withdrawn several millimeters.
- Once pericardial fluid is aspirated, disconnect the syringe from the needle and thread a J wire through the needle (see **Figure 4-2** and **Figure 4-3**).

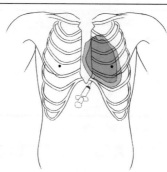

FIGURE 4-1. Subxiphoid Approach to Pericardiocentesis

Pericardiocentesis needle is inserted 1 cm below and to the left of the xiphoid notch directed toward the left shoulder.

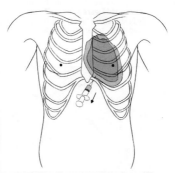

FIGURE 4-2. Aspiration of Pericardial Fluid

Pericardial fluid is aspirated. In equivocal cases, pericardial fluid can be differentiated from blood because it does not clot.

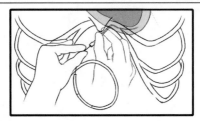

FIGURE 4-3. Threading Wire Through the Needle

Once pericardial fluid is aspirated, the syringe is disconnected and a flexible wire is advanced through the needle. The needle is then withdrawn leaving the wire in place.

- Remove the needle and leave the wire in place
- Make a 3-mm skin incision along the wire using a scalpel
- Introduce dilator over the wire and then remove the dilator, leaving the wire in place (**Figure 4-4**).
- Introduce the drainage catheter over wire until it is within the pericardial space, then remove the wire and secure the catheter in place with suture (see **Figure 4-5** and **Figure 4-6**).
- Manually aspirate fluid or attach the catheter to a sterile drainage bag
- Obtain a postprocedure electrocardiogram, echocardiogram, and chest x-ray

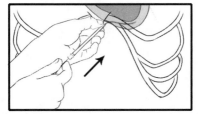

FIGURE 4-4. Advancing Dilator Over Wire

A dilator is advanced over the wire to dilate a soft tissue tract into the pericardium.

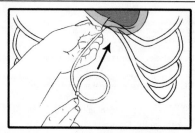

FIGURE 4-5. Pericardiocentesis Catheter Is Introduced Over Wire

A pericardiocentesis catheter is advanced over wire to an appropriate depth of insertion.

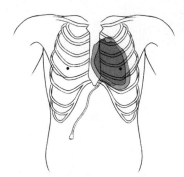

FIGURE 4-6. Pericardiocentesis Catheter In Place

After the pericardiocentesis catheter is introduced, the wire is withdrawn and the pericardiocentesis catheter is secured in place.

WORK-UP OF PERICARDITIS

- **Blood work**: Complete blood count, renal panel, troponin I; ANA, rheumatoid factor, TSH and PPD skin test.
- **Pericardial Fluid Analysis**
  - Routine studies: cell count and differential, protein, glucose, lactate dehydrogenase, pH, cultures and gram stain
  - Optional studies: cultures for fungi and acid-fast bacilli, AFB RNA by PCR, adenosine deaminase level and cytology

CODING

33010	Pericardiocentesis, initial
33011	Pericardiocentesis, subsequent
76930	Ultrasound guidance for pericardiocentesis

REFERENCES

Mayo Clin Proc. 2002; 77: 429.
Curr Treatment Options Cardiovasc Med. 1999; 1: 79.
Clin Cardiology. 2008; 31: 531–537.
Canadian J Cardiol. 1999; 15: 1251.
Intensive Care Med. 2000; 26: 573.
NEJM. 2004; 351: 2195.

5 ■ SYNCHRONIZED CARDIOVERSION

INDICATIONS

- Unstable supraventricular tachyarrhythmia with a pulse (atrial fibrillation, atrial flutter, or reentrant tachycardia)
  - Signs of instability: angina; depressed level of consciousness; heart failure; or hypotension
  - Clinical instability is unlikely to be secondary to a tachyarrhythmia if the ventricular rate is less than 150 beats/min.
- Unstable wide complex tachycardia (ventricular tachycardia or supraventricular tachycardia with aberrancy) with a pulse
- New-onset atrial fibrillation/flutter within the past 48 hours
- Refractory ventricular tachycardia with a pulse

CONTRAINDICATIONS TO ELECTIVE CARDIOVERSION

- Absent pulse
- Electrolyte abnormalities
- Presence of a left atrial or left ventricular thrombus
- Insufficient anticoagulation for patients in chronic atrial fibrillation/flutter
- Digitalis toxicity
- Atrial fibrillation > 6 months or associated with a left atrial diameter > 4.5 cm (relative)
- Sick sinus syndrome without an implanted pacemaker

EQUIPMENT

- Cardioversion device with electrode pads or paddles
  - Biphasic devices are superior to monophasic devices.
- Conductive gel or patches (if paddles used)
- Airway management equipment (bag-valve mask, supplemental oxygen, laryngoscope with various blades, endotracheal tube, oral airway, and suction equipment)
- ACLS medications
- Cardiac monitor with appropriate leads and electrodes
- Pulse oximeter and blood pressure monitor

TECHNIQUE

- No food or liquids for at least six hours (elective cardioversion).
- Place patient in supine position.
- Continuous cardiac monitoring and pulse oximetry.
- Select a lead with prominent R waves (usually lead II) to avoid "R on T" phenomenon.
- Secure a large-bore peripheral IV line.
- Apply electrode pads in either the anterolateral or the anterior-posterior position (see **Figure 5-1** and **Figure 5-2**).
    - Alternatively, paddle electrodes can be used with conductive gel in the anterolateral position.
    - Avoid placement of pads/paddles within 5 inches of any internal pacemaker, monitor electrodes, or transdermal patches.
    - Anterior-posterior pad position has a higher success rate compared with the anterolateral position.
- Recommend procedural sedation to a level of moderate sedation (see Chapter 1) with one of the following:
    - Etomidate 0.15 mg/kg IV over 30 seconds
    - Midazolam 0.05 mg/kg IV every two–three minutes titrated to effect (max. 0.15 mg/kg)
    - Propofol 1–1.5 mg/kg IV over 30 seconds
    - Fentanyl 0.5–1 mcg/kg IV (added as an adjunct if more sedation needed)

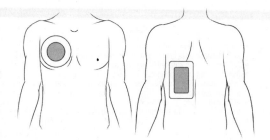

FIGURE 5-1. Placement of Anterior-Posterior Pads For Synchronized Cardioversion
Adapted from Shea JB, Maisel WH. Cardioversion. *Circulation*. 2002; 106(22): e177, Figure 1.

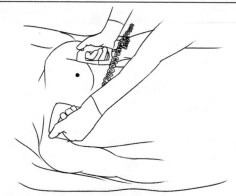

FIGURE 5-2. Cardioversion Using Paddles In Anterolateral Position

- Select synchronized mode on cardioverter.
- Select energy level (**Table 5-1**).
- Ensure that all personnel are clear of the bed and patient.
- Deliver shock.
- Evaluate patient's cardiac rhythm, vital signs, and level of consciousness.
- If unsuccessful, increase the energy level with consecutive shocks.

TABLE 5-1. Recommended Initial Energy Levels for Synchronized Cardioversion

Rhythm	Energy Levels (Joules)	
	Monophasic	Biphasic
Atrial flutter	50	50
Atrial fibrillation	100	100
Supraventricular tachycardia	50	50
Monomorphic ventricular tachycardia	100	50
Polymorphic ventricular tachycardia	200	100

Source: Data from American Heart Association. 2005 Guidelines on Electrical Therapies, Part 5: Electrical Therapies: Automated External Defibrillators, Defibrillation, Cardioversion, and Pacing. *Circulation*. 2005; 112: IV-35–IV-46.

COMPLICATIONS

- Respiratory depression (from sedatives)
- Hypotension (from sedatives)
- Bradycardia
- Ventricular tachycardia
- Ventricular fibrillation (from "R on T" phenomenon)
- Asystole
- Skin burns (especially if inadequate conductive gel used)
- Stroke
- Myocardial infarction
- Chest pain (if inadequate procedural sedation given)

CODING

92960   Cardioversion, external

REFERENCES

Am Heart J. 2005; 149: 316–321.
Am Heart J. 2005; 150: 150–152.
Acad Emerg Med. 2001; 8: 545.
Heart. 2002; 88: 117–118.
Amer J Cardiol. 2000; 86: 348–350.

6 ■ TRANSCUTANEOUS PACING

INDICATIONS

- Bradyarrhythmia with hemodynamic instability unresponsive to atropine
- Temporary stabilization of Mobitz type II second-degree AV block, sinus arrest, or complete heart block
- May be considered in witnessed asystolic cardiac arrest (within the first few minutes) refractory to medications

CONTRAINDICATIONS

- Severe hypothermia
- Awake, hemodynamically stable patients
- Non-intact skin at the electrode site
- Ventricular fibrillation

EQUIPMENT

- Supplemental oxygen by nasal cannula or face mask
- Suction apparatus with Yankauer suction tip
- Bag valve mask
- Intubation supplies (laryngoscope, endotracheal tubes, stylet, oral airways, tape, end-tidal CO_2 detector)
- Pacing electrode pads
- ECG electrodes for rhythm monitoring
- Combined pacemaker/cardiac monitor/defibrillator unit

TECHNIQUE

- Administer supplemental oxygen.
- Remove excess hair in the areas of pacer pad placement.
- Apply anterior-posterior or anterolateral pacing pads and connect leads to pacemaker (**Figure 6-1**).
- Place patient on a cardiac monitor.
- Strongly consider an analgesic/anxiolytic for conscious patients.
- Turn pacemaker to "pacing mode."
- Select pacing mode (demand [or synchronous mode] vs fixed [or asynchronous mode]).
  * Demand pacing is recommended (this mode paces only when the spontaneous heart rate falls below the level set by the physician).

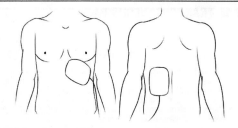

FIGURE 6-1A. Placement of Anterior-Posterior Pads for Transcutaneous Pacing
Adapted from Shea JB, Maisel WH. Cardioversion. *Circulation.* 2002; 106(22): e177, Figure 1.

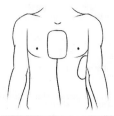

FIGURE 6-1B. Placement of Anterolateral Pads for Transcutaneous Pacing
Adapted from Gammage MD. Temporary Cardiac Pacing. *Heart.* 2000; 83(6): 718, Figure 3.

- Set the desired pacer rate (typically 60 beats/min).
- Start the pacemaker at 0 mA (milliamps) for conscious patients (**Figure 6-2A**).
  - For asystolic or unconscious patients, start at 200 mA and gradually decrease.
- In conscious patients, gradually increase the output by 5–10-mA increments until the pacemaker captures (pacer spikes are seen in front of every wide QRS complex) (**Figure 6-2B**).
- Slowly decrease the output to the lowest level that maintains capture; keep the output level ~10% higher than this minimum level.

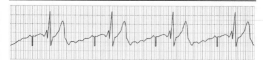

FIGURE 6-2A. Rhythm Strip With Pacing Spikes and No Capture

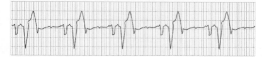

FIGURE 6-2B. Rhythm Strip Demonstrating Good Pacing Capture

COMPLICATIONS

- Ventricular dysrhythmias
- Skin burns
- Chest wall discomfort during pacing (minor)

CODING

92953   Transcutaneous pacing

REFERENCES

Ann Emerg Med. 1989; 18: 1280–1286.
J Emerg Med. 1985; 2: 155–162.
Ann Emerg Med. 1986; 15: 121–124.
N Engl J Med. 1983; 309: 1166–1168.
Crit Care Med. 1990; 18: 572–573.
J Emer Med. 2007; 32: 105–111.
Bessman, E. Emergency Cardiac Pacing. In: Roberts JR, Hedges JR, eds.
      Clinical Procedures in Emergency Medicine. 5th ed. Philadelphia, PA:
      Saunders; 2009: 282–286.

SECTION IV

DERMATOLOGY PROCEDURES

7 ■ LACERATION REPAIR

INDICATIONS

- Repair of wounds < 12 hours old on trunk or extremities; < 24 hours old on the face or scalp
- Delayed primary closure of wounds after three–five days of wound-packing
- Consider for small animal bite wounds to the face or scalp

CONTRAINDICATIONS

- Large human or animal bite wounds
- Wounds > 12 hours on trunk or extremities; > 24 hours on the face or scalp
- Puncture or deep-penetrating wounds
- Grossly infected wounds
- Grossly contaminated wounds, farm cuts, or wounds with a high risk of contamination
  - Leave open if > 6 hours since injury

EQUIPMENT

- Surgical prep (povidone-iodine or chlorhexidine)
- 60-ml syringe with 18-gauge angiocatheter
- Sterile bowl filled with normal saline
- 1% lidocaine +/− epinephrine
- 3–5-ml syringe with an 18-gauge needle
- 27-gauge needle, 1 ¼-inch
- Sterile drape
- 4 × 4-inch gauze sponges
- Needle holder
- Iris scissors
- Hemostat
- Suture scissors
- Adson forceps with teeth
- Scalpel with No. 15 blade
- Appropriate suture(s)
- Electrocautery unit
- Sterile gloves
- Mask with face shield

TECHNIQUE

- Perform a careful neurovascular exam.
- Consider an x-ray for any possibility of an underlying fracture or retained foreign body.
- Assess need for tetanus prophylaxis
- Copious wound irrigation with normal saline using a 60-ml syringe connected to an 18-gauge angiocatheter; use 50–100-ml irrigant for each cm of wound size.
- Remove additional debris with forceps.
- Sharp debridement of devitalized tissue or irregular edges with a scalpel or tissue scissors.
- Sterile prep of surrounding skin.
- Anesthetize wound edges with 1% lidocaine +/– epinephrine.
  - Avoid epinephrine for digits, nose, penis, or earlobes.
  - Minimize discomfort by using a 27-gauge needle, inject slowly, warm solution, and buffer solution with 8.4% sodium bicarbonate (1 ml bicarbonate per 10 ml lidocaine).
- If the wound margins close with too much tension, undermine wound edges at the dermal-adipose junction as far back as the wound is wide, using scissors, scalpel, or electrocautery.
- Assure hemostasis using pressure or electrocautery prior to wound closure.
- Close dead space with deep stitches and inverted knots using absorbable suture (e.g., Vicryl, Dexon, or Monocryl) (**Figure 7-1**).
- Skin is closed with careful approximation of wound edges and minimal skin tension.
- Options for skin closure using nonabsorbable suture (e.g., nylon, Prolene, Plain Gut [for face] or Surgilene):
- **Simple interrupted suture (Figure 7-2)**
  - Suture is as wide as it is deep
  - Symmetric on both sides
  - Skin margins slightly everted
- **Simple running suture (Figure 7-3)**
  - Keep spacing and depth of suture equal on both sides.
  - Distributes tension evenly.
- **Vertical mattress suture (Figure 7-4)**
  - Promotes skin eversion
  - Best for posterior neck, loose skin, or concave skin surfaces
- **Horizontal mattress suture (Figure 7-5)**
  - Best for wounds under tension (e.g., finger lacerations over joints) or for very thin skin
  - Promotes skin eversion
- **Tissue adhesives (e.g., Dermabond) (Figure 7-6)**
  - For areas of low skin tension (e.g., face, shin, dorsal hand).
  - Avoid if patient at risk for poor wound healing and if laceration on eyebrow or scalp.

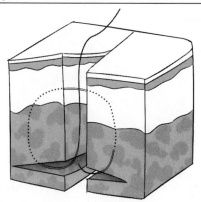

FIGURE 7-1. Deep Interrupted Suture With Buried Knot
Adapted from Zuber TJ. Fusiform Excision. *Amer Fam Physician*. 2003; 67(7): 1541, Figure 3.

The depth of suture placement should be symmetrical on both sides.

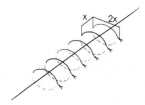

FIGURE 7-2. Simple Interrupted Suture
Adapted from Forsch RT. Essentials of Skin Laceration Repair. *Amer Fam Physician*. 2008; 78(8): 948, Figure 1A.

The depth of suture placement should be symmetrical on both sides.

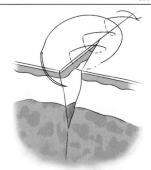

FIGURE 7-3. Running Stitch
Adapted from Forsch RT. Essentials of Skin Laceration Repair. *Amer Fam Physician.* 2008; 78(8): 948, Figure 1B.

The depth of suture placement and the degree of advancement should remain constant.

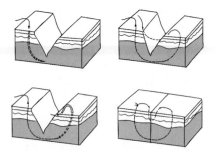

FIGURE 7-4. Vertical Mattress Suture
Adapted from Forsch RT. Essentials of Skin Laceration Repair. *Amer Fam Physician.* 2008; 78(8): 948, Figure 3.

Initially, the wound is entered and exited a generous distance from the wound edges. The suture is then re-entered and exited 1–2 mm from the wound edge. The depth of suture placement should be symmetrical on both sides.

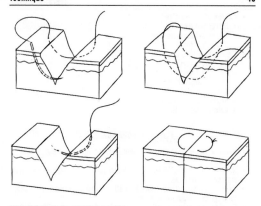

FIGURE 7-5. Horizontal Mattress Suture
Adapted from Forsch RT. Essentials of Skin Laceration Repair. *Amer Fam Physician*. 2008; 78(8): 948, Figure 4.

The depth of suture placement should be identical for all needle passes. Also, the distance from the wound edge should remain constant.

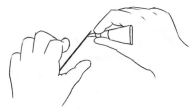

FIGURE 7-6. Proper Technique For the Application of Tissue Adhesive In Laceration Repair
Adapted from Forsch RT. Essentials of Skin Laceration Repair. *Amer Fam Physician*. 2008; 78(8): 949, Figure 6.

The thumb and index finger push the wound edges together while the tissue adhesive is applied.

- **Choice of suture size**
  - 3-0 or 4-0 for trunk
  - 4-0 or 5-0 for extremities
  - 5-0 or 6-0 for face
- **Timing of suture removal**
  - Face: 4–5 days
  - Neck: 5–7 days
  - Hand or arms: 7–10 days
  - Trunk: 10–14 days
  - Scalp, feet, or legs: 10–14 days
  - Palms or soles: 14–21 days

POSTPROCEDURE CARE

- Apply a three-layer dressing: nonadherent dressing (e.g., Adaptic), gauze, and tape or roll.
- Remove dressing in 48 hours and leave open to air; keep wound clean with soap and water.
- Td or Tdap if last vaccination was > 10 years for any wound or > 5 years for large or contaminated wounds.
- Consider prophylactic antibiotics × 5 days for: patients with diabetes, peripheral vascular disease, malnutrition, morbid obesity, alcoholism, or renal failure; immunocompromised patients; human and animal bites; crush injuries; penetrating injuries; or wounds over a joint or with a high degree of contamination with soil or debris.

COMPLICATIONS

- Wound infection
- Bleeding or wound hematoma
- Wound dehiscence
- Unrecognized damage to internal structures: tendons, nerves, muscles, or blood vessels
- Keloids or hypertrophic scar formation

CODING

TABLE 7-1. CPT Codes for Laceration Repairs

Location	Length (cm)	CPT Code
Simple Repairs		
Trunk, scalp, or extremities	≤ 2.5	12001
	2.6–7.5	12002
	7.6–12.5	12004
Face, ears, or eyelids	≤ 2.5	12011
	2.6–5	12013
	5.1–7.5	12014
Intermediate Repairs		
Trunk, scalp, or extremities	≤ 2.5	12031
	2.6–7.5	12032
	7.6–12.5	12034
Neck, hands, or feet	≤ 2.5	12041
	2.6–7.5	12042
	7.6–12.5	12044
Face, ears, or eyelids	≤ 2.5	12051
	2.6–5	12052
	5.1–7.5	12053

Source: Data from *CPT 2007.* Chicago, IL: American Medical Association; 2006.

REFERENCES

Amer Fam Physician. 2008; 78: 945–951.
Emer Med Clin N Amer. 2007; 25: 73–81.
NEJM. 2006; 355: e18.
MMWR Recommendation Rep. 1991; 40 (RR-10): 1–28.

8 ■ CRYOSURGERY OF SKIN LESIONS

INDICATIONS

- Benign skin lesions: acrocordon (skin tags); cherry angiomas; condyloma acuminata; cutaneous horns; dermatofibromas; granuloma annulare; hypertrophic scars; keloids; milia; molluscum contagiosum; papular nevi; pyogenic granulomas; sebaceous hyperplasia; seborrheic keratoses; solar lentigo; and viral warts
- Actinic keratoses
- Bowen's disease (squamous cell carcinoma in-situ)
- Superficial basal cell carcinoma

CONTRAINDICATIONS

- Melanoma
- Areas with compromised circulation
- Recurrent skin cancer
- Sclerosing basal cell carcinoma
- Need for histopathologic exam of skin lesion
- Caution with treatment in a hair-bearing area, or periorbital, nasolabial fold, ala nasi, or eyelid margin areas
- Relative contraindications: cryoglobulinemia; cold urticaria; Raynaud's disease; Collagen-vascular disease; Pyoderma gangrenosum; heavily pigmented skin; or multiple myeloma

EQUIPMENT

- Liquid nitrogen in storage container
- Liquid nitrogen spray gun **OR**
- Liquid nitrogen bottle with cryoprobe **OR**
- Styrofoam cup and cotton-tipped applicator

TECHNIQUE FOR LIQUID NITROGEN SPRAY GUN OR CRYOPROBE (FIGURE 8-1)

- Select appropriate nozzle size for liquid nitrogen spray gun.
  - Hold nozzle 1–2 cm from target and direct spray directly on the skin lesion until an ice ball is created.

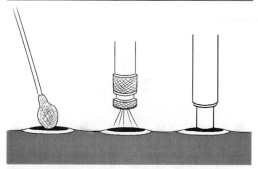

FIGURE 8-1. Cryosurgery Devices
Adapted from Andrews MD. Cryosurgery for Common Skin Conditions. *Amer Fam Physician*. 2004; 69(10): 2365, Figure 1.

(Left) Cotton-tip applicator. (Center) Liquid nitrogen spray. (Right) Cryoprobe.

- Also, various sizes of cryoprobes can attach to the liquid nitrogen spray container.
  - Place cryoprobe directly on lesion and freeze with the liquid nitrogen spray gun.
- Freeze times:
  - Benign lesions require an ice ball 2 mm beyond the lesion (**Figure 8-2**).
  - Premalignant lesions require an ice ball 2–3 mm beyond the lesion (see **Figure 8-2**).
  - Malignant lesions require an ice ball 5 mm beyond the lesion.

TECHNIQUE FOR Q-TIP APPLICATION (SEE FIGURE 8-1)

- Partially fill a styrofoam cup with liquid nitrogen.
- Use a Q-tip for small lesions or a large cotton-tipped swab for large lesions.
- Dip the swab into the liquid nitrogen; then touch the center of the lesion with the swab.
- Periodically dip applicator into liquid nitrogen; treat lesion until freeze is complete.

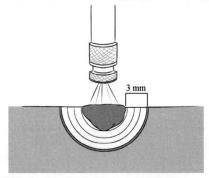

FIGURE 8-2. Cryosurgery Technique Used to Create an Ice Ball
Adapted from Andrews MD. Cryosurgery for Common Skin Conditions. *Amer Fam Physician.* 2004; 69(10): 2367, Figure 5.

Cryosurgery creates an ice ball between 3–5 mm around a skin lesion.

POSTPROCEDURE CARE

- Keep area clean.
- Apply an antibiotic or petrolatum ointment to wounds once or twice daily.

COMPLICATIONS

- Excessive cryotherapy can cause skin necrosis, but rarely scars.
- Blistering or skin ulcer formation.
- Hypopigmentation or hyperpigmentation.
- Hair loss.

CODING

11200	Removal of skin tags, 1–15 lesions
11201	Skin tags, each additional 10 lesions
17000	Destruction of premalignant lesions; first lesion

17003	As for 17000, premalignant lesions 2–14
17004	As for 17000, ≥ 15 premalignant lesions treated
17110	Destruction of benign skin lesions other than skin tags or vascular lesions; up to 14 lesions
17111	As for 17110, 15 or more lesions
17260	Destruction malignant lesion trunk, arm or leg ≤ 0.5 cm
17261	Destruction malignant lesion trunk, arm or leg 0.6–1 cm
17262	Destruction malignant lesion trunk, arm or leg 1.1–2 cm
17270	Destruction malignant lesion scalp, neck, hands, feet, or genitalia ≤ 0.5 cm
17271	Destruction malignant lesion scalp, neck, hands, feet, or genitalia 0.6–1 cm
17272	Destruction malignant lesion scalp, neck, hands, feet, or genitalia 1.1–2 cm
17280	Destruction malignant lesion face, ears, eyelids, nose, lips, or mucous membranes ≤ 0.5 cm
17281	Destruction malignant lesion face, ears, eyelids, nose, lips, or mucous membranes 0.6–1 cm
17282	Destruction malignant lesion face, ears, eyelids, nose, lips, or mucous membranes 1.1–2 cm
46916	Anal or perianal, benign lesion, simple cryosurgery
46924	Anal or perianal, benign lesion, extensive cryosurgery
54056	Penis, benign lesion, simple cryosurgery
54065	Penis, benign lesion, extensive cryosurgery
56501	Destruction of lesion(s), vulva, simple cryosurgery
56515	Destruction of lesion(s), vulva, extensive cryosurgery
67850	Destruction of lesion of eyelid or lid margin (up to 1 cm)

Adapted from *Current Procedural Terminology: CPT 2002*. Standard ed. Chicago, IL: American Medical Association; 2001:48, 56, 144, 161, 167, 199.

REFERENCES

Amer Fam Physician. 2004; 69: 2365–2372.
Amer Fam Physician. 2005; 72: 845–848.
Amer Fam Physician. 2004; 70: 1481–1488.
Can Fam Physician. 1999; 45: 964–974.

9 ■ SHAVE SKIN BIOPSY

INDICATIONS

- Removal of skin lesions that appear benign
- Removal of basal cell carcinomas
- Removal of low-risk squamous cell carcinomas < 2 cm in size
- Rashes of unclear etiology

CONTRAINDICATIONS

- Subcutaneous lesions
- Any pigmented lesion (may be a melanoma)
- Infection at planned biopsy site
- Coagulopathy (relative contraindication)

EQUIPMENT

- Sterile prep (povidone-iodine or chlorhexidine)
- Sterile gloves
- 1% lidocaine +/− epinephrine
- 3-ml syringe with 27-gauge needle
- Flexible razor blade or scalpel (No. 10 or 15)
- Monsel's (ferric subsulfate) solution or 35% aluminum chloride solution
- Antibiotic ointment
- Sterile bandage
- Specimen container
  - with formalin for routine histopathology
  - with saline for tissue culture

TECHNIQUE

- Sterile prep of area.
- Anesthetize skin within the dermis using 1% lidocaine +/− epinephrine to raise the skin lesion above the surrounding skin (**Figure 9-1**).
  - Avoid epinephrine for digits, nose, penis, or earlobes.
  - Minimize discomfort by using a 27-gauge needle, injecting slowly, and buffering solution with 8.4% sodium bicarbonate (1 ml bicarbonate per 10 ml lidocaine).
- Excise lesion with a blade.
  - Razor blade is slightly bowed and pushed laterally under skin lesion in one uninterrupted motion (**Figure 9-2**).

- • Scalpel blade is kept parallel to the surrounding skin and lesion excised at its base with a straight lateral motion or with a cutting motion (**Figure 9-3**).
- • Apply pressure to the wound.
- • Apply Monsel's solution or 35% aluminum chloride on the wound to achieve hemostasis.
- • Apply a sterile Band-aid.

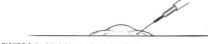

FIGURE 9-1. Administering Local Anesthesia
Adapted from Grekin RC, Auletta MJ. Local anesthesia in dermatologic surgery. *J Amer Acad Dermatol.* 1988; 19(4): 603, Figure 4.

Lidocaine is injected under the skin lesion to elevate the lesion above the surrounding skin.

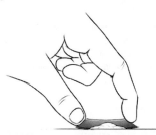

FIGURE 9-2. Shave Biopsy of Skin Lesion Using a Razor Blade
Adapted from Alguire PC, Mathes BM. Skin Biopsy Techniques for the Internist. *J Gen Intern Med.* 1998; 13(1): 49, Figure 2.

Tension is applied to each side of a razor blade to create a slight curvature. The blade is then passed beneath the lesion to remove it at the dermal level.

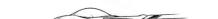

FIGURE 9-3. Shave Biopsy of Skin Lesion Using a Scalpel

A scalpel is passed beneath the skin lesion to remove it at the dermal level.

POSTPROCEDURE CARE

- Keep wound covered for 24 hours.
- Apply an antibiotic or petrolatum ointment to wounds once or twice daily

COMPLICATIONS

- Infection
- Bleeding
- Scarring or hypopigmentation
  - Occurs more commonly if the shave biopsy was too deep

CODING

11100	Skin biopsy of one lesion
11101	Skin biopsy, each additional lesion
11755	Biopsy of nail
41100	Biopsy of tongue lesion, anterior two thirds
41105	Biopsy of tongue lesion, posterior one third
54100	Biopsy of penile skin lesion
56605	Biopsy of first vulvar or perineal lesion
56606	Biopsy of vulvar or perineal lesion, each additional lesion
57100	Biopsy of vagina, simple
67810	Biopsy of eyelid
69100	Biopsy of pinna

REFERENCES

J Amer Acad Derm. 2005; 52: 516–517.
J Gen Intern Med. 1998; 13: 46–54.
J Family Practice. 2003; 52: 210–218.
Amer Fam Physician. 1996; 54: 2411.
Cutis. 1994; 53: 172–186.

10 ■ EXCISIONAL SKIN BIOPSY

INDICATIONS

- Removal of any benign or potentially malignant skin lesion
- Removal of nevi
- Removal of subcutaneous lesions

CONTRAINDICATIONS

- Infection at planned biopsy site
- Coagulopathy (relative contraindication)

EQUIPMENT

- Surgical prep (povidone-iodine or chlorhexidine)
- 1% lidocaine +/− epinephrine
- 5-ml syringe with an 18-gauge needle
- 27-gauge needle, 11/4 inch
- Sterile drape
- 4 × 4-inch gauze sponges
- Sterile marking pen
- Needle holder
- Iris scissors
- Hemostat
- Suture scissors
- Adson forceps with teeth
- Scalpel with No. 15 blade
- Appropriate suture(s)
- Electrocautery unit
- Sterile gloves
- Mask with face shield
- Specimen container
  - with formalin for routine histopathology
  - with saline for tissue culture

TECHNIQUE

- Area is prepped and draped.
  - Use extreme caution in the areas of the "deadly triangles": the glabella, sternum, and mid-upper back. These areas are particularly

difficult to close without tension and are prone to stria and keloid formation.

- Use pen to draw an elliptical margin around skin lesion with the long axis oriented parallel to the body's skin tension lines [Lines of Langer] (see **Figure 10-1** and **Figure 10-2**).
  - Length of ellipse is 3 times its width.
- Anesthetize wound edges with 1% lidocaine +/− epinephrine.
  - Avoid epinephrine for digits, nose, penis, or earlobes.
  - Minimize discomfort by using a 27-gauge needle, injecting slowly, and buffering solution with 8.4% sodium bicarbonate (1 ml bicarbonate per 10 ml lidocaine)
- Make an incision through the dermis with a scalpel along the outlined ellipse (**Figure 10-3**).
- Elevate one corner of ellipse with forceps and excise the lesion with a scalpel from the corner to the center. Repeat this step from other corner (**Figure 10-4**).
- Place the skin lesion in a specimen container.
- Assure hemostasis using pressure or electrocautery prior to wound closure.
- If the wound margins close with too much tension, two options are available:
  - Undermine wound edges bilaterally as far back as the wound is wide using tissue scissors, scalpel, or electrocautery.
  - Close subcutaneous tissue with deep stitches and inverted knots using absorbable suture (e.g. Vicryl, Dexon, or Monocryl) (see **Figure 7-1, p 41**).
- Skin is closed with careful approximation of wound edges and minimal skin tension.
- Options for skin closure using nonabsorbable suture (e.g., nylon, Prolene, or Surgilene):
  - Simple interrupted suture (see **Figure 7-2, p 41**)
  - Simple running suture (see **Figure 7-3, p 42**)
  - Vertical mattress suture (see **Figure 7-4, p 42**)
  - Horizontal mattress suture (see **Figure 7-5, p 43**)
- **Choice of suture size**
  - 3-0 or 4-0 for trunk
  - 4-0 or 5-0 for extremities
  - 5-0 or 6-0 for face
- **Timing of Suture Removal**
  - Face: 4–5 days
  - Neck: 5–7 days
  - Hand or arms: 7–10 days
  - Trunk: 10–14 days
  - Scalp, feet, or legs: 10–14 days
  - Palms or soles: 14–21 days

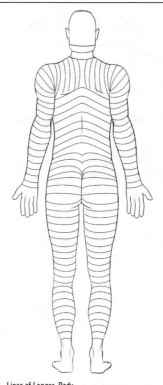

FIGURE 10-1. Lines of Langer: Body
Adapted from Zuber TJ and Mayeaux EJ. *Atlas of Primary Care.* Philadelphia, PA: Lippincott Williams & Wilkins; 2004: 95, Figure 1B.

Fusiform excisions should parallel the Lines of Langer, which outline the lines of least skin tension. These lines run perpendicular to the lower torso and the long axis of the extremities.

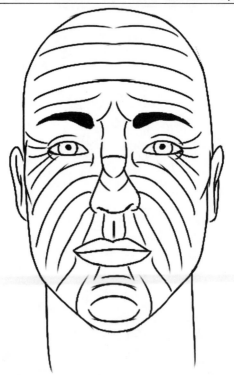

FIGURE 10-2. Lines of Langer: Face
Adapted from Zuber TJ and Mayeaux EJ. *Atlas of Primary Care.* Philadelphia, PA: Lippincott
Williams & Wilkins; 2004: 95, Figure 1C.

Fusiform excisions should parallel the Lines of Langer, which outline the lines
of least skin tension.

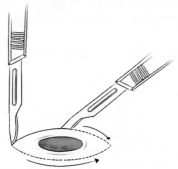

FIGURE 10-3. Elliptical Incision Around Skin Lesion
Adapted from Reynolds PL, Strayer SM. Treatment of Skin Malignancies. *J Fam Practice*, 2003; 52(6): 458, Figure 2.

Make an elliptical incision 3 times longer than the ellipse is wide.

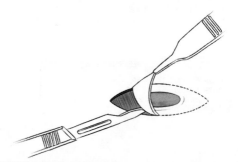

FIGURE 10-4. Excising the Skin Lesion
Adapted from Salam GA. Lipoma Excision. *Amer Fam Physician*. 2002; 65(5): 902, Figure 3.

Grasp the corner of the skin island with Adson forceps and undermine the skin with a scalpel in the subcutaneous fat.

POSTPROCEDURE CARE

- Apply an antibiotic or petrolatum ointment to wounds repaired by suture 1–2 times daily.

COMPLICATIONS

- Wound infection
- Bleeding or wound hematoma
- Wound dehiscence

CODING

11100	Skin biopsy of one lesion
11101	Skin biopsy, each additional lesion
11755	Biopsy of nail
41100	Biopsy of tongue lesion, anterior two thirds
41105	Biopsy of tongue lesion, posterior one third
54100	Biopsy of penile skin lesion
56605	Biopsy of first vulvar or perineal lesion
56606	Biopsy of vulvar or perineal lesion, each additional lesion
57100	Biopsy of vagina, simple
67810	Biopsy of eyelid
69100	Biopsy of pinna

REFERENCES

J Gen Intern Med. 1998; 13: 46–54.
J Family Practice. 2003; 52: 210–218.
Amer Fam Physician. 1996; 54: 2411.
Patient Care. 2001; 30: 11.

11 ■ PUNCH SKIN BIOPSY

INDICATIONS

- Evaluation of suspected skin tumors
- Evaluation of bullous skin disorders
- Evaluation of any abnormal skin lesion
- Removal of small skin lesions

CONTRAINDICATIONS

- Not appropriate for subcutaneous lesions
- Acutely infected sites
- Skin lesions directly over tendons, ligaments, nerves, or arteries
- Coagulopathy or bleeding diathesis (relative)

COMPLICATIONS

- Infection
- Bleeding
- Keloid formation

EQUIPMENT

- Various sizes of biopsy instruments (trephines): 2 mm, 3 mm, 4 mm, 5 mm, or 6 mm
- 1% lidocaine with epinephrine
- 3-ml syringe
- 1 1/4-inch 21-gauge and 27-gauge needles
- Antisepsis: Chlorhexidine or povidone-iodine swabs
- Jar of 10% formalin
- Sterile gloves
- Needle holder
- 4-0 or 5-0 nylon suture
- Iris scissors
- Sterile bandage

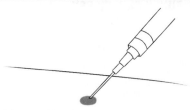

FIGURE 11-1. Anesthetizing Skin
Adapted from Grekin RC, Auletta MJ. Local anesthesia in dermatologic surgery. *J Amer Acad Dermatol.* 1988; 19(4): 603, Figure 4.

The skin is anesthetized with 1% lidocaine under the skin lesion.

TECHNIQUE

- Clean biopsy site with antiseptic solution.
- Anesthetize skin lesion with 1% lidocaine with epinephrine (**Figure 11-1**).
- The thumb and index finger of the nondominant hand are used to stretch the skin perpendicular to the lines of least skin tension (which correspond to the long axis of the legs or arms).
- The trephine is placed vertically over the skin lesion and advanced downward with a twisting motion until the instrument penetrates the subcutaneous fat (see **Figure 11-2**).
- Remove the trephine and elevate the skin lesion using the anesthesia needle.
- Excise the skin lesion at the base using Iris scissors (**Figure 11-3**).
- Place a simple interrupted suture perpendicular to Lines of Langer to close the wound (**Figure 11-4**).
- Cover wound with a bandage

CODING

11100	Biopsy of skin, subcutaneous
11101	Biopsy of each additional lesion (must be reported with 11100)

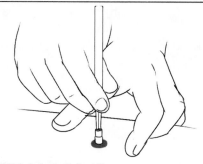

FIGURE 11-2. Performing the Punch Biopsy
Adapted from Zuber TJ. Punch Biopsy of the Skin. *Amer Fam Physician*. 2002; 65(6): 1157, Figure 2A.

A punch biopsy instrument is advanced through the skin lesion with a rotating motion until the instrument hub reaches the skin.

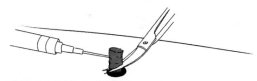

FIGURE 11-3. Excising the Skin Biopsy
Adapted from Zuber TJ. Punch Biopsy of the Skin. *Amer Fam Physician*. 2002; 65(6): 1157, Figure 2B.

The skin biopsy is elevated with a needle and excised at the base with Iris scissors.

FIGURE 11-4. Closing Biopsy Incision
Adapted from Zuber TJ. Punch Biopsy of the Skin. *Amer Fam Physician*. 2002; 65(6): 1156, Figure 1C.

The resulting incision is closed with a simple interrupted suture.

REFERENCES

Am Fam Physician. 2002; 65: 1155–1158.

J Gen Intern Med. 1998; 13: 46–54.

Usatine RP, Moy RL, Tobinick EL, et al. *Skin Surgery: A Practical Guide*. St Louis, MO: Mosby; 1998: 101–119.

Consultant. 1994; 34: 1167–1168.

INDICATIONS

- Ingrown toenails (onychocryptosis) refractory to conserva...
  management
- Refractory onychomycosis
- Onychogryposis (deformed, curved nail)
- Chronic, recurrent paronychia (inflamed nail fold)

CONTRAINDICATIONS

- Infected toe (except for paronychia with surrounding cellulitis)
- Poor vascular inflow to digit (relative)
- Coagulopathy (relative)
- Avoid phenol use during pregnancy

EQUIPMENT

- Sterile prep (providone-iodine or chlorhexidine)
- Sterile gloves
- 10-mL syringe with 27-gauge needle
- 1% lidocaine
- Small penrose drain or donut tourniquet (optional)
- Narrow Locke periosteal elevator
- English anvil nail splitter
- Sterile scissors with straight blade
- Two straight hemostats
- Dermal curette
- 4 × 4-inch sterile gauze pack
- Small gauze roll
- Several silver nitrate sticks
- Antibiotic ointment
- Cotton-tipped applicators
- 88% phenol solution if permanent nail ablation planned
- 70% isopropyl alcohol (isopropanol)

TECHNIQUE

- prep of affected toe
- dminister a digital nerve block **(Figure 12-1)**.
- Introduce needle transversely across base of the toe, dorsal aspect
  - Inject 1 mL 1% lidocaine as needle withdrawn
- Insert needle vertically through anesthetized skin at base of toe adjacent to bone until it tents the volar skin; withdraw needle slightly then inject 1 mL 1% lidocaine; inject an additional 1 mL anesthetic as needle withdrawn.
- Repeat procedure on medial and lateral side of toe.
- May apply donut tourniquet or use a Penrose drain secured in place with hemostat at base of digit.
- Lift the side of the nail with a periosteal elevator; advance under the proximal nail fold; separate 1/3 of nail from nail bed **(Figure 12-2)**.
- Use nail splitter to split nail past the cuticle **(Figure 12-3)**.
- Grasp nail with a hemostat and remove by twisting outward toward the lateral nail fold **(Figure 12-4)**.
- Remove excess granulation tissue using a dermal curette or scissors **(Figure 12-5)**.
- Apply silver nitrate to nail bed until good hemostasis
  - For nail matrix ablation, apply 88% phenol to nail matrix for 30 seconds × 3 using a cotton-tipped applicator; then neutralize phenol with 70% isopropanol **(Figure 12-6)**.

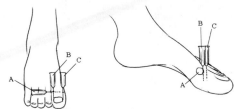

FIGURE 12-1. Digital Block of Toe
Adapted from Williams JG, Lalonde DH. Randomized Comparison of the Single-Injection Volar Subcutaneous Block and the Two-Injection Dorsal Block for Digital Anesthesia. *Plast Reconstruct Surg.* 2006; 118(5): 1196, Figure 1.

All injections use 1% lidocaine at the base of the toe. The first injection is along the dorsum of the toe (A); then two columns of anesthesia are created along the sides of the toe (B and C) at the level of the first webspace. A—Front View; B—Side View.

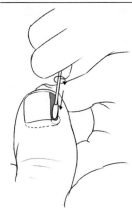

FIGURE 12-6. Nail Ablation With Phenol
Adapted from Heidelbaugh JJ, Lee H. Management of the Ingrown Toenail. *Amer Fam Physician.* 2009; 79(4): 307, Figure 8.

A cotton applicator is used to ablate the nail matrix with phenol.

- Indications for matrix ablation: recurrent paronychia; severe acute paronychia; or paronychia associated with diabetes, peripheral vascular disease, Raynaud's syndrome, or an immunocompromised state.
- Remove tourniquet and apply antibiotic ointment and gauze pressure dressing.

POSTPROCEDURE CARE

- Keep foot elevated and remove dressing in 24 hours.
- Wash toe several times daily.
- Trim toenails straight and not too short.

COMPLICATIONS

- Recurrent ingrown toenail
- Infection (rare)
- Bleeding

CODING

11730	Nail removal, partial or complete
11750	Permanent nail removal (matrixectomy), partial or complete

REFERENCES

Amer Fam Physician. 2009; 79: 303–308.
Clin Podiatr Med Surg. 2004; 21: 617–630.
Cochrane Database Syst Rev. 2005; (2): CD001541.
Cutis. 2006; 78(6): 407–408.
Can Fam Physician. 1988; 34: 2675–2681.

13 ■ INCISION AND DRAINAGE OF ABSCESSES

- Drainage of any symptomatic cutaneous abscess
  - Classic features of an abscess include rubor, dolor, tumor, and calor.

CONTRAINDICATIONS

- Abscesses that may require extensive debridement under general anesthesia
  - Perirectal abscess, perineal abscess, or hand abscess
  - Deep abscesses involving the face, neck, feet, axillae, or groin areas

EQUIPMENT

- Sterile gloves
- Sterile towels or fenestrated drape
- Protective gown and eyewear
- 1% lidocaine +/− epinephrine
- 10-ml and 20-ml syringes
- 14-gauge angiocatheter
- 25-gauge needle
- Skin prep: chlorhexidine or povidone-iodine swabs
- Scalpel with a No. 11 blade
- Curved hemostats
- Plain or iodoform packing gauze
- Culture tube
- 4 × 4-inch sterile gauze pads
- Tape

TECHNIQUE

- Soft tissue x-ray if there is any concern for a retained foreign body (e.g., needle or glass fragments).
- Sterile prep of the abscess and surrounding skin.
- Sterile drape of the area.
- Anesthesia options: regional block; field block by infiltrating the skin circumferentially around the abscess; or local anesthesia of the skin

69

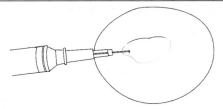

FIGURE 13-1. Anesthesia for Incision and Drainage

Local anesthetic is injected to anesthetize the skin overlying the abscess.

overlying abscess; use of 1% lidocaine with sodium bicarbonate (mixed in 1:10 ratio) reduces the injection pain (**Figure 13-1**).
  - Consider procedural sedation for abscesses in sensitive areas, large abscesses, or for patient anxiety (see Chapter 1).
- Make a linear incision with a scalpel, covering the entire width of the abscess following the Lines of Langer (see **Figure 13-2**, **Figure 10-1** [p **55**], and **Figure 10-2** [p **56**]).
- Culture the purulent material extruded from the wound.
- Probe the abscess cavity in all directions with a hemostat to break up any remaining loculations (**Figure 13-3**).
- Irrigate large abscess cavities with normal saline using a 20-ml syringe attached to a 14-gauge angiocather.

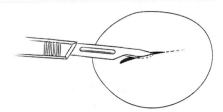

FIGURE 13-2. Scalpel Incision of Abscess Wall
Adapted from Fitch MT, Manthey DE, McGinnis HD, et al. Abscess Incision and Drainage. *N Engl J Med.* 2007; 357(18): e22, Figure 3.

A scalpel is used to create a generous incision into the abscess cavity.

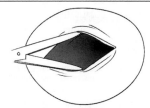

FIGURE 13-3. Blunt Dissection to Break up Loculations Within the Abscess Cavity
Adapted from Fitch MT, Manthey DE, McGinnis HD, et al. Abscess Incision and Drainage. *N Engl J Med.* 2007; 357(18): e22, Figure 4.

A hemostat is used to break up the loculations within the abscess cavity.

- Pack the wound loosely with packing gauze in order to keep the incision open (**Figure 13-4**).
- Apply sterile 4 × 4-inch gauze over wound and tape in place.
- Change the packing gauze every 24–48 hours until the wound has an established drainage tract and the base has healthy granulation tissue.
- At this point, perform daily wet-to-dry saline dressing changes until the wound is completely healed.
- Indication for antibiotics: hemodynamic instability, surrounding cellulitis, immunocompromised patients, or those at high risk for developing endocarditis (prosthetic heart valve, prior infective endocarditis, cardiac transplant, and some patients with a history of congenital heart disease).

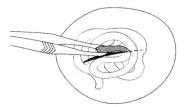

FIGURE 13-4. Packing Abscess Cavity
Adapted from Fitch MT, Manthey DE, McGinnis HD, et al. Abscess Incision and Drainage. *N Engl J Med.* 2007; 357(18): e22, Figure 5.

The abscess cavity is packed with packing gauze leaving a tail outside the skin.

COMPLICATIONS

- Procedural pain
- Abscess recurrence
- Fistula formation
- Bleeding
- Necrotizing fasciitis (if an inadequate wound-debridement is performed)
- Damage to surrounding nerves, vessels, and lymphatics
- Keloid formation

CODING

10060	Incision and drainage of single abscess or simple abscess
10061	Incision and drainage of multiple abscesses or complex abscess
10080	Incision and drainage of simple pilonidal cyst
10140	Incision and drainage of hematoma
10180	Incision and drainage of complex, post-operative wound infection
21501	Incision and drainage of deep neck or thoracic abscess
23030	Incision and drainage of deep shoulder abscess
23930	Incision and drainage of deep upper arm or elbow abscess
25028	Incision and drainage of deep forearm or wrist abscess
27301	Incision and drainage of deep thigh or knee abscess
27603	Incision and drainage of deep lower leg or ankle abscess
28002	Incision and drainage of deep foot abscess
40801	Incision and drainage of complicated mouth abscess
55100	Incision and drainage of scrotal wall abscess
56405	Incision and drainage of vulvar or perineal abscess
69000	Incision and drainage of pinna abscess, simple
69005	Incision and drainage of pinna abscess, complex

REFERENCES

J Am Acad Dermatol. 2004; 51: 132.
Circulation. 2007; 116: 1736.
Ann Emerg Med. 2007; 50: 49–51.
Ann Emerg Med. 1985; 14: 15.
JACEP. 1978; 7: 186.
NEJM. 2007; 357: e20.
Amer Fam Physician. 2005; 72: 2474–2481.
Am J Surg. 1978; 135: 721.

14 ■ LIPOMA OR SUBCUTANEOUS MASS EXCISION

INDICATIONS

- Excision of lipoma or subcutaneous mass

CONTRAINDICATIONS

- Masses at high risk for malignancy should be excised in the operating room (size > 5 cm, associated calcifications, invading adjacent structures).
- Overlying skin infection.
- Coagulopathy or bleeding diathesis (relative).

COMPLICATIONS

- Wound infection
- Hematoma
- Seroma formation
- Nerve injury
- Excessive scarring with tissue contracture or deformity
- Keloid formation
- Periostitis/osteomyelitis

EQUIPMENT

- Skin-marking pen
- No. 15 scalpel blade with handle
- Antiseptic solution: chlorhexidine or povidone-iodine swabs
- Needle holder
- Metzenbaum scissors
- Iris scissors
- Adson forceps
- Two hemostats
- Allis clamp
- Pack of sterile 4 × 4-inch gauze
- Tape
- Fenestrated drape
- 10 ml 1% lidocaine with epinephrine
- 10-ml syringe

- 1-inch 18-gauge and 1.5-inch 27-gauge needles
- 3-0 Chromic or Vicryl suture
- 4-0 or 5-0 nylon suture
- Jar of 10% formalin

ENUCLEATION TECHNIQUE FOR SMALL LIPOMAS

- Prep the skin with an antiseptic solution and cover the area with a fenestrated drape.
- Anesthetize the skin using 1% lidocaine with epinephrine to create a field block.
- Make a small linear incision across the center of the lipoma (**Figure 14-1**).
- Dissect down and around the lipoma with scissors or a hemostat (**Figure 14-2**).

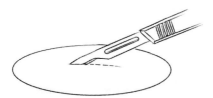

FIGURE 14-1. Linear Incision Over Lipoma
Adapted from Pfenninger JL, Fowler GC, eds. *Procedures for Primary Care*. Philadelphia, PA: Elsevier; 2011: 77, Figure 12-15A.

A linear incision is made with a scalpel over the middle of the lipoma.

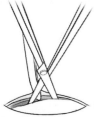

FIGURE 14-2. Lysing Adhesions Around Lipoma
Adapted from Pfenninger JL, Fowler GC, eds. *Procedures for Primary Care*. Philadelphia, PA: Elsevier; 2011: 77, Figure 12-15B.

Scissors or a curved hemostat are used to dissect around the lipoma.

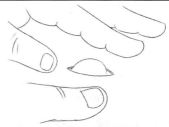

FIGURE 14-3. Expressing Lipoma Through Skin Incision

Adapted from Pfenninger JL, Fowler GC, eds. *Procedures for Primary Care*. Philadelphia, PA: Elsevier; 2011: 77, Figure 12-15D.

Lateral finger pressure elevates the lipoma into the skin incision.

- Enucleate the lipoma using lateral finger pressure to elevate the lipoma into the skin incision (**Figure 14-3**).
- Grasp the lipoma with an Allis clamp and excise the mass at its base using iris scissors.
- Use interrupted nylon sutures to close the incision.

EXCISION TECHNIQUE FOR LARGE LIPOMAS OR SUBCUTANEOUS MASSES

- Draw an elliptical outline to guide your skin incision, with the width about 2/3 the diameter of the subcutaneous mass and the length 3 times longer than the width.
  - The long axis of the fusiform exision should follow Lines of Langer (**Figure 10-1** [p 55] and **Figure 10-2** [p 56]).
- Prep the skin with an antiseptic solution and cover the area with a fenestrated drape.
- Anesthetize the skin using 1% lidocaine with epinephrine to create a field block.
- Incise the skin with a scalpel along the fusiform outline (**Figure 14-4**).
- Grasp the island of skin with an Allis clamp.
- Metzenbaum scissors or a scalpel are used to undermine the lateral skin and dissect through the subcutaneous fat to the lipoma while pulling traction with the Allis clamp (**Figure 14-5**).
- Once the bulk of the lipoma has been dissected away from the surrounding tissue, a gloved finger can sweep around the lesion and deliver it through the skin incision.

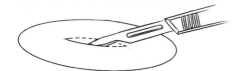

FIGURE 14-4. Initial Elliptical Incision Over Lipoma
Adapted from Salam GA. Lipoma Excision. *Amer Fam Physician*. 2002; 65(5): 902, Figure 3.

A fusiform skin incision is made over the middle of the lipoma.

- Excise the mass at its base using iris scissors.
- Deep buried interrupted Chromic or Vicryl sutures are placed to close the dead space (see **Figure 7-1**, p **41**)
- Use interrupted nylon sutures to close the incision (see **Figure 7-2**, p **41**)
- Apply a gauze pressure dressing for 48 hours.

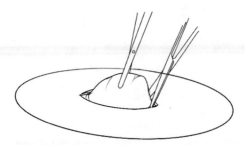

FIGURE 14-5. Sharp Dissection Around Sides of Lipoma
Adapted from Salam GA. Lipoma Excision. *Amer Fam Physician*. 2002; 65(5): 903, Figure 4.

Scissors are used to dissect around the lipoma while traction is applied using an Allis clamp.

CODING

11400	Benign excision trunk-arm-leg < 0.6 cm
11401	Benign excision trunk-arm-leg 0.6–1 cm
11402	Benign excision trunk-arm-leg 1.1–2 cm
11403	Benign excision trunk-arm-leg 2.1–3 cm
11404	Benign excision trunk-arm-leg 3.1–4 cm
11406	Benign excision trunk-arm-leg > 4 cm
11420	Benign excision scalp-neck-hands-feet-genitalia < 0.6 cm
11421	Benign excision scalp-neck-hands-feet-genitalia 0.6–1 cm
11422	Benign excision scalp-neck-hands-feet-genitalia 1.1–2 cm
11423	Benign excision scalp-neck-hands-feet-genitalia 2.1–3 cm
11424	Benign excision scalp-neck-hands-feet-genitalia 3.1–4 cm
11426	Benign excision scalp-neck-hands-feet-genitalia > 4 cm

REFERENCES

Mayeaux EJ. *The Essential Guide to Primary Care Procedures*. Philadelphia, PA: Lippincott Williams & Wilkins; 2009: 386–393.

Amer Fam Physician. 2002; 65: 901–904.

Bennett RG. *Fundamentals of Cutaneous Surgery*. St. Louis, MO: Mosby; 1988: 726–731.

Brit J Surg. 1995; 82 (12): 1649–50.

Pfenninger JL, Fowler GC, eds. *Procedures for Primary Care*. Phildelphia, PA: Elsevier; 2011: 76–77.

SECTION V

EAR, NOSE, AND THROAT PROCEDURES

15 ■ TYMPANOMETRY

INDICATIONS

- Evaluation of hearing impairment
- Evaluation of unexplained vertigo or Eustachian tube dysfunction
- Assess for middle ear effusions
- Assess tympanic membrane compliance

CONTRAINDICATIONS

- Otorrhea or ear bleeding
- Otitis externa
- External auditory canal injury or obstruction

COMPLICATIONS

- External auditory canal abrasions

EQUIPMENT

- Tympanometer with printer
- Probe covers

TECHNIQUE

- Otoscopy should be performed to visualize the external auditory canal and tympanic membrane.
- Gently pull the helix of the ear posterosuperiorly.
- Insert the tympanometry probe into the external auditory canal and create a tight seal.
- Activate the tympanometer to obtain pressure readings (i.e., tympanograms).
- Print a record of the tympanogram (**Figure 15-1**).

CODING

92567   Tympanometry

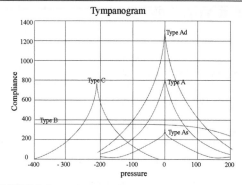

FIGURE 15-1. Tympanograms
Adapted from Mayeaux EJ. *The Essential Guide to Primary Care Procedures.* Philadelphia, PA:
Lippincott Williams & Wilkins; 2009: 787, Figure 1.

Type A tympanogram is normal; Type Ad occurs with a highly compliant tympanic membrane with a low impedance; Type As occurs when the tympanic membrane has decreased compliance (e.g., otosclerosis); Type B is a flat tympanogram suggesting a middle ear effusion; Type C has a high compliance peak in the negative pressure range (e.g., Eustachian tube dysfunction).

REFERENCES

Feldman AS and Wilber LA. *Acoustic Impedance and Admittance: The Measurement of Middle Ear Function.* Baltimore, MD: Lippincott Williams & Wilkins; 1976: 103.
Mayeaux EJ. *The Essential Guide to Primary Care Procedures.* Philadelphia, PA: Lippincott Williams & Wilkins; 2009: 787–790.
Pediatrics. 2004; 113: 1412–1429.
Pediatrics. 2006; 118: 1–13.
Amer Fam Physician. 2004; 70: 1713–1720.

16 ■ INTRANASAL DEVICE PLACEMENT FOR EPISTAXIS

- Anterior epistaxis
- Posterior epistaxis

CONTRAINDICATIONS

- Basilar skull fracture
- Massive facial trauma
- Cerebrospinal fluid leak
- Septal hematoma

EQUIPMENT

- Gloves, mask with face shield, and gown
- Chair or gurney with a headrest
- Nasal speculum
- Headlamp or other good light source
- Local anesthetic and vasoconstrictor: 4% cocaine is the preferred solution
  - Alternatives: 1% tetracaine mixed 1:1 with 0.05% oxymetazoline (Afrin); or 0.5% phenylephrine (Neo-Synephrine) mixed 2:1 with 4% lidocaine
- Bayonet forceps
- Suction device with a Frazier tip catheter
- Cotton-tipped swabs
- Cotton pledgets
- Silver nitrate sticks
- 4 × 4-inch gauze
- 5% viscous lidocaine
- 5-mL syringe
- 10-mL vial sterile saline or sterile water
- Tape
- Emesis basin
- Intranasal balloon device or nasal tampon

TECHNIQUE

- Check for thrombocytopenia or a coagulopathy.
  - Indications for a platelet transfusion: platelets $< 50,000/mm^3$ or clopidogrel use and severe epistaxis
  - Indications for fresh frozen plasma: INR > 1.5 or PTT $> 1.5 \times$ upper limit of normal and severe epistaxis
- Control hypertension.
- Have the patient in a sitting position with the base of the nose parallel to the floor.
- The patient should blow his/her nose to remove any clots.
- Soak a cotton pledget in the local anesthetic/vasoconstrictor solution (**Figure 16-1**).
- Fill the affected nostril with soaked cotton pledgets (up to three) using a Bayonet forceps and leave in place for 4–5 minutes (**Figure 16-2**).
  - Have the patient squeeze the affected nostril during this period.
- Remove the cotton pledgets and inspect the nostril using a nasal speculum.
- If a distinct area of bleeding is identified in Kiesselbach's plexus, roll silver nitrate sticks over the affected mucosa to cauterize the area.
  - Gently apply petroleum jelly using a cotton-tipped swab over the cauterized area.
- If cautery is unsuccessful or if no obvious source of persistent epistaxis is identified, place an intranasal device.
  - Select options for anterior epistaxis: Rhino Rocket; Epi-Stop Balloon Catheter; Rapid Rhino; Rapid-Pac; Merocel nasal tampon; or a Merocel Doyle nasal pack
  - Merocel tampon placement (**Figure 16-3**)
    - Spread 5% viscous lidocaine on Merocel nasal tampon.
    - Insert nasal tampon 2 cm into nares leaving strings outside the nose.
    - Rehydrate tampon with 5 ml sterile saline.
  - Balloon catheter placement (e.g., Rhino Rocket, Epi-Stop, or Rapid-Pac balloon catheters) (**Figure 16-4**)
    - Catheter may need to be soaked in sterile water for 30 seconds (Rhino Rocket).
    - Fully insert balloon catheter parallel to the floor of nasal cavity.

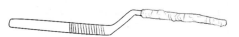

FIGURE 16-1. Cotton Pledget

Adapted from Roberts JR, Hedges JR, eds. *Clinical Procedures in Emergency Medicine.* 5th ed. Philadelphia, PA: Saunders; 2009: 1199, Figure 64-30B.

This cotton pledget was soaked in vasoconstricting solution and will be inserted into the nares using a bayonet forceps.

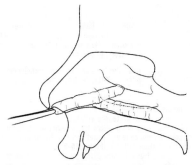

FIGURE 16-2. Placement of Cotton Pledgets Into Nasal Cavity
Adapted from Roberts JR, Hedges JR, eds. *Clinical Procedures in Emergency Medicine.* 5th ed. Philadelphia, PA: Saunders; 2009: 1199, Figure 64-30D.

Cotton pledgets are inserted into the nares to anesthetize the nasal cavity. Typically, 2–3 pledgets are placed to accomplish this.

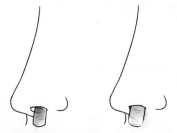

FIGURE 16-3. Placement of Merocel Tampons
Adapted from Roberts JR, Hedges JR, eds. *Clinical Procedures in Emergency Medicine.* 5th ed. Philadelphia, PA: Saunders; 2009: 1205, Figure 64-37C.

A dehydrated Merocel tampon is lubricated with 5% viscous lidocaine and then the full length is inserted into the nose (A). Saline is used to expand the tampon such that it expands to fit securely into the nasal cavity (B).

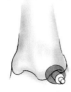

FIGURE 16-4. Balloon Catheter in Place

Adapted from Roberts JR, Hedges JR, eds. *Clinical Procedures in Emergency Medicine.* 5th ed. Philadelphia, PA: Saunders; 2009: 1208, Figure 64-40C.

This patient has had a balloon catheter device placed within his left nares for control of epistaxis.

- Inflate balloon with air or saline.
- Secure balloon cuff to face with tape.
- Select dual-balloon catheters for posterior epistaxis or epistaxis of unknown source (e.g., Epistat catheter; Nasostat catheter; or an Epi-Max Balloon Catheter) **(Figure 16-5)**
  - Fully insert dual-balloon device parallel to the floor of the nasal cavity.
  - Slowly inflate the posterior balloon with 7–10 ml air or saline.
  - Withdraw device until posterior balloon seats itself in the posterior nasal cavity.
  - Slowly inflate the anterior balloon with 15–30 ml air or saline **(Figure 16-6)**.
    - Stop balloon inflation if acute pain develops
- Remove nasal packs after three–five days.
- Consider prophylactic antibiotics with amoxicillin or trimethoprim/sulfamethoxazole while nasal packing is in place.
- Avoid NSAIDs and salicylate-containing products for at least five days.

COMPLICATIONS

- Sinusitis
- Nasopharyngeal tissue necrosis
- Dysphagia

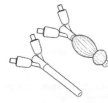

FIGURE 16-5. Dual Balloon Nasal Catheters

Adapted from Roberts JR, Hedges JR, eds. *Clinical Procedures in Emergency Medicine.* 5th ed. Philadelphia, PA: Saunders; 2009: 1208, Figure 64-40A.

Dual-balloon catheters can serve as both an anterior and a posterior pack for control of either anterior or posterior epistaxis. (A) Deflated catheter; (B) Inflated catheter.

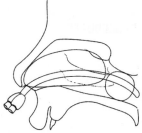

FIGURE 16-6. An Inflated Dual-Balloon Catheter In Position
Adapted from Roberts JR, Hedges JR, eds. *Clinical Procedures in Emergency Medicine.* 5th ed. Philadelphia, PA: Saunders; 2009: 1208, Figure 64-40B.

Cross-section of the nasal cavity demonstrating the proper position of an inflated dual-balloon catheter.

- Eustachian tube dysfunction
- Dislodgement of intranasal device
- Septal perforation (very rare)
- Toxic shock syndrome (very rare)

CODING

30901	Control anterior epistaxis, simple, any method
30903	Control anterior epistaxis, complex, any method
30905	Control posterior epistaxis with posterior nasal packs, any method, initial
30906	Control posterior epistaxis with posterior nasal packs, any method, subsequent

REFERENCES

J Oral Maxillofacial Surg. 2000; 58: 419.
Ann Emerg Med. 2005; 45: 134.
Amer Fam Physic. 2005; 71: 305.
Otolaryngol Clin N Amer. 2008; 41: 525.
NEJM. 2009; 360: 784.
Roberts JR, Hedges JR, eds. *Clinical Procedures in Emergency Medicine,* 5th ed. Philadelphia, PA: Saunders; 2009: 1199–1208.

SECTION VI

GASTROINTESTINAL PROCEDURES

17 ■ PARACENTESIS

INDICATIONS

- **Diagnostic Paracentesis**
  - Evaluate etiology of new-onset ascites
  - Rule out spontaneous bacterial peritonitis
  - Follow-up of therapy for spontaneous bacterial peritonitis (not mandatory)
- **Therapeutic Paracentesis**
  - Respiratory compromise in patients with massive ascites
  - Management of refractory, cirrhotic ascites
  - Adjunctive management of hepatorenal syndrome

CONTRAINDICATIONS

- **Absolute contraindications**
  - Acute abdomen requiring exploratory surgery
  - Infected abdominal wall at the entry site
  - Uncooperative patient
  - Disseminated intravascular coagulation or fibrinolysis
- **Relative contraindications**
  - Severe bowel distension or bowel obstruction
  - Multiple prior abdominal surgeries
  - Pregnancy
  - Coagulopathy with PTT $\geq 2\times$ upper limit of normal
  - Thrombocytopenia (platelets < 50K)

EQUIPMENT

- Chlorhexidine or povidone-iodine swabs
- 5-ml syringe and needles for anesthesia
- 1% lidocaine +/− epinephrine
- 18-gauge angiocatheter, 3 inches; or 3 1/4-inch Caldwell needle
- 50–60-ml syringe for aspirating ascitic fluid
- Three-way stopcock
- High-pressure drainage tubing (e.g., blood-collection tubing)
- Several large-volume evacuated containers for therapeutic paracentesis

TECHNIQUE

- Informed Consent.
- Perform a "time out" to assure correct patient and correct procedure.
- Position: Consider use of ultrasound to confirm a good fluid pocket; assure that patient remains in the same position for paracentesis.
  - Semi-recumbent and flat for midline approach (**Figure 17-1**).
    - Insertion site is 2–3 cm inferior to umbilicus.
  - Semi-recumbent and left lateral tilt for left lower quadrant approach (see **Figure 17-1**)
    - Insertion site is 4–5 cm toward the umbilicus from the anterior superior iliac spine and lateral to rectus muscle.
- Sterile prep and drape.
- Local anesthesia of skin and subcutaneous tissue to peritoneum.
- Z tract method until peritoneal fluid obtained; then advance catheter over needle (**Figure 17-2**).
  - Retract skin cephalad while inserting the paracentesis needle perpendicular to the skin until there is return of ascitic fluid; then release traction.
- Collect 50 ml of ascitic fluid for diagnostic tests (**Figure 17-3**).
- Connect drainage tubing to an evacuated container for a therapeutic paracentesis (**Figure 17-4**).

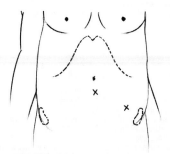

FIGURE 17-1. Paracentesis Insertion Sites
Adapted from Thomsen TW, Shaffer RW, White B, et al. Paracentesis. *N Engl J Med.* 2006; 355(19): e22, Figure 1.

A midline insertion site is 2–3 cm below the umbilicus. A left lower quadrant insertion site is 4–5 cm toward the umbilicus from the anterior superior iliac spine.

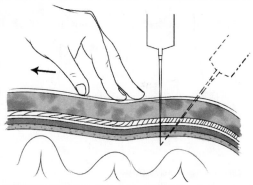

FIGURE 17-2. Z Tract Method for Insertion of a Paracentesis Needle
Adapted from Thomsen TW, Shaffer RW, White B, et al. Paracentesis. *N Engl J Med.* 2006;
355(19): e22, Figures 3A and 3B.

Apply traction on skin as the needle is introduced perpendicular to skin
(solid syringe); once ascitic fluid is aspirated, traction is released (dashed
syringe).

WHEN TO USE ALBUMIN

- Consider if preexisting renal insufficiency (creatinine > 1.2 mg/dl)
- Hepatorenal syndrome
- Presence of spontaneous bacterial peritonitis
  - 1.5 gm/kg IV on day 1 and then 1 gm/kg IV on day 3
  - 23% absolute risk reduction of renal impairment and 19% absolute
    reduction in 90-day mortality for albumin vs. placebo (p = 0.01)
- Postprocedure hypotension
- Controversial if needed prophylactically for paracentesis of > 5–6
  liters
  - 6–8 gm albumin for every 1 liter removed above 5–6 liters ascitic
    fluid

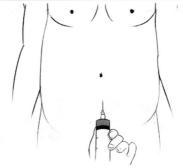

FIGURE 17-3. Aspiration of Ascitic Fluid

A 3 1/4-inch Caldwell needle is inserted until ascitic fluid is aspirated. Then the blunt metal catheter is advanced over the needle and left in place as the needle is withdrawn.

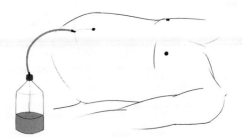

FIGURE 17-4. Therapeutic Paracentesis Using an Evacuated Container

Collection tubing is connected on one end to the paracentesis catheter and on the other end to an evacuated container during a therapeutic paracentesis.

TABLE 17-1. Ascitic Fluid Classification

Serum-ascites albumin gradient ≥ 1.1 gm/d	Serum-ascites albumin gradient < 1.1 gm/dl
Cirrhotic ascites	Peritoneal carcinomatosis
Alcoholic hepatitis	Peritoneal tuberculosis
Right-sided CHF	Pancreatic ascites
Multiple liver metastases	Biliary ascites
Fulminant hepatic failure	Nephrotic syndrome
Budd-Chiari syndrome	Lupus serositis
Portal vein thrombosis	Bowel infarction/obstruction
Veno-occlusive disease	Postoperative lymphatic leak
Fatty liver of pregnancy	
Myxedema	

ASCITIC FLUID ANALYSIS (TABLE 17-1)

- Routine studies: cell count and differential; protein; lactate dehydrogenase; glucose; albumin; gram stain and bedside inoculation of aerobic and anaerobic culture bottles
- Optional studies if clinically indicated: amylase; triglycerides; cytology; AFP culture; AFB RNA by PCR and adenosine deaminase level
- Serum-ascites albumin gradient (SAAG) = difference between serum and ascitic fluid albumin
  - The SAAG is used to classify ascitic fluid (**Table 17-2**).

COMPLICATIONS

- **Major Complications**
  - Bowel or bladder perforation
  - Laceration of aorta or mesenteric, iliac, or inferior epigastric arteries
    - Risk of major hemorrhagic complication 1–2%
  - Sheared-off catheter fragment
  - Hypotension with large volume paracentesis
  - Hepatorenal syndrome with large volume paracentesis

TABLE 17-2. Ascitic Fluid Analysis

EDTA-treated tube	Comments
Cell count and differential*	≥ 250 PMN/mm³ = SBP; WBC ≥ 17,000 = secondary bacterial peritonitis
Aerobic/anaerobic cultures	Innoculate culture bottles at bedside for best yield
Tube without additives	
Total protein*	≥ 1 gm/dl suggests secondary bacterial peritonitis
Lactate dehydrogenase (LDH)*	Suggests secondary bacterial peritonitis if less than upper limit of normal for serum
Glucose*	< 50 mg/dl suggests secondary bacterial peritonitis
Albumin	SAAG = serum albumin—ascitic fluid albumin
Amylase	> 2000 U/liter if hollow viscus perforation or pancreatic ascites
Triglycerides	> 200 mg/dl suggest chylous ascites
Carcinoembryonic antigen (CEA)	> 5 ng/dl suggests hollow viscus perforation
Alkaline phosphatase	≥ 240 U/liter suggests hollow viscus perforation
Syringe or evacuated container	
Cytology	Sensitivity improved if 3 samples submitted and promptly evaluated
AFB culture	Sensitivity = 50%
AFB RNA by PCR	Sensitivity = 85%; Specificity = 99%

* Secondary becterial peritonitis suggested if ascitic fluid has WBC>=17,000; polymicrobial gram stain; or 2 of the following 3 abnormalities: protein >=1 gm/dL; LDH>225 Units/mL; glucose <50mg/dL.

- **Minor Complications**
  - Persistent ascitic fluid leak (can fix with interrupted skin suture)
  - Metastatic seeding of needle tract
  - Soft-tissue infection at puncture site
  - Abdominal wall hematoma

CODING

49080	Abdominal paracentesis, initial
49081	Abdominal paracentesis, subsequent

REFERENCES

NEJM. 2006; 355: e21–e24.
NEJM. 1999; 341: 403–409.
Hepatology. 2004; 39: 841–856.
Amer J Gastroenterol. 2006; 101: 1954–1955.
JAMA. 1978; 239: 628–630.

SECTION VII

GENITOURINARY PROCEDURES

18 ■ NO-SCALPEL VASECTOMY

INDICATIONS

- Permanent sterilization

CONTRAINDICATIONS

- Scrotal infection or epididymo-orchitis
- Inability to palpate and elevate both vasa
- Lack of a firm desire for permanent sterility
- Coagulopathy or clopidogrel use (relative)
- Large inguinal hernia or varicocele (relative)

EQUIPMENT

- Sterile prep (povidone-iodine or chlorhexidine)
- Two Vas-fixing forceps (Vas clamps)
- Sharp dissecting forceps
- Two hemostats
- Adson forceps
- Iris scissors
- Surgical clip applicator
- 4 medium stainless steel surgical clips; or 3-0 Vicryl suture ties
- Thermal cautery unit
- 10-ml syringe with a 1 1/2-inch 25-gauge needle
- 1% lidocaine
- 0.5% bupivacaine
- 4 × 4-inch sterile gauze pack
- Sterile fenestrated drape
- Sterile gloves
- Specimen jar with formalin
- Needle holder and 4-0 Vicryl suture

TECHNIQUE

- Assure that the special vasectomy consent forms have been signed and that the waiting period requirement has been met.
- Consider premedication with diazepam 5 mg PO 30 minutes prior to procedure.
- Patient in supine position with legs together.
- Place the penis underneath a sterile drape to keep it out of the sterile field.

- Shave scrotum of any hair.
- Warm sterile prep of scrotum.
- Sterile drape of area.
- Move vas to the midline raphe and grasp with a three-finger technique (**Figure 18-1**).
- Anesthetize scrotal skin over vas with 1:1 mixture of 1% lidocaine/0.5% bupivicaine using a 25-gauge needle (**Figure 18-2A**).
- Advance needle 2 cm parallel and adjacent to vas; inject 2–4 ml anesthetic mixture (see **Figure 18-2B**).
- Withdraw the needle slightly, and then re-advance 180° around the vas and inject another 2–4 mL of anesthetic mixture.
- Grasp vas through anesthetized skin with a vas clamp (**Figure 18-3**).
- Use sharp dissecting forceps to spread scrotal tissue ~5 mm and dissect down to vas.
- Stab vas with one jaw of the dissecting forceps through the scrotal incision.
- Rotate dissecting forceps so the jaws are pointing upward to elevate the vas.
- Grasp exposed vas with a vas clamp and elevate vas through incision.
- Use dissecting forceps to strip perivas fascia and further isolate vas (**Figure 18-4**).
- Grasp perivas fascia proximally with two hemostats to isolate a 1.5-cm segment of vas.

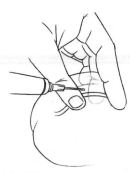

FIGURE 18-1. Holding Vas

Adapted from Clenney TL, Higgins JC. Vasectomy Techniques. *Amer Fam Physician.* 1999; 60(1): 142, Figure 3.

Three-finger grasp of vas deferens.

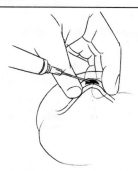

FIGURE 18-2A. Anesthesia of Vas
Adapted from Clenney TL, Higgins JC. Vasectomy Techniques. *Amer Fam Physician.* 1999; 60(1): 140, Figure 2A.

Injection of lidocaine directly over the vas.

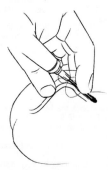

FIGURE 18-2B. Anesthesia of Vas
Adapted from Clenney TL, Higgins JC. Vasectomy Techniques. *Amer Fam Physician.* 1999; 60(1): 140, Figure 2B.

Paravasal injection of lidocaine after 2.5 cm advancement of needle in cephalic direction.

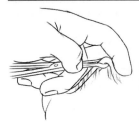

FIGURE 18-3. Grasping Vas
Adapted from Li SQ, Goldstein M, Zhu J, et al. The no-scalpel vasectomy. *J Urol.* 1991; 145(2): 342, Figure 2B.

The vas is grasped through scrotum with vasectomy clamp and elevated.

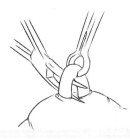

FIGURE 18-4. Stripping of Perivas Fascia
Adapted from Clenney TL, Higgins JC. Vasectomy Techniques. *Amer Fam Physician.* 1999; 60(1): 144, Figure 8.

Use dissecting forceps to strip away perivas fascia; then puncture the perivas fascia with jaws closed directly underneath vas; then open jaws to widen the opening.

- Place two surgical clips (or use 4-0 Vicryl suture) on each side of vas under hemostats (**Figure 18-5**).
- Excise 1-cm segment of vas above hemostats and place in specimen jar (**Figure 18-6**).
- Insert cautery tip 5 mm into the vas lumen and cauterize the vas on both ends (**Figure 18-7**).
- Place a purse-string suture using 4-0 Vicryl to close the fascia over the prostatic end of vas (Fascial Interposition).
  * The fascia must be closed below the cut testicular end of the vas.
- Close scrotal incision with 4-0 Vicryl buried interrupted sutures.
- Use pack of 4 × 4-inch gauze under scrotum and hold in place with a scrotal support.
- Place an ice pack next to the scrotum immediately.

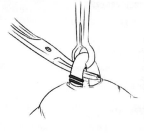

FIGURE 18-5. Ligating the Isolated Vas

Adapted from Clenney TL, Higgins JC. Vasectomy Techniques. *Amer Fam Physician.* 1999; 60(1): 146, Figure 9.

Apply two medium surgical clips on each side of the isolated vas using a surgical clip applicator (or vas can be ligated using 3-0 Vicryl suture).

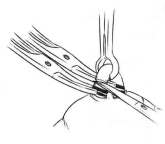

FIGURE 18-6. Excising a Segment of the Vas

Adapted from Dassow P, Bennett JM. Vasectomy: An Update. *Amer Fam Physician.* 2006; 74(12): 2072, Figure 1A.

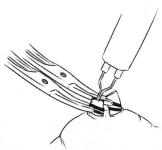

FIGURE 18-7. Cauterizing the Ends of the Vas

Adapted from Clenney TL, Higgins JC. Vasectomy Techniques. *Amer Fam Physician.* 1999; 60(1): 148, Figure 10.

POSTPROCEDURE CARE

- Wear scrotal support for 2–3 days.
- Ice scrotal area for 12 hours.
- Keep scrotum dry for 48 hours.
- No heavy lifting or strenuous exercise × 1 week.
- Avoid sexual intercourse for 1 week.
- Alternative birth control until semen analysis negative.
- Semen analysis after 6–8 weeks or 15 ejaculations.
  - Repeat semen analysis after 3 months.

COMPLICATIONS

- Hematoma: minor hematomas are common; need for reexploration is rare
- Sperm granuloma (rare)
- Infection of scrotal skin or epididymis (approximately 1%)
- Congestive epididymitis
- Post-vasectomy pain syndrome

CODING

55250	Vasectomy
89321	Semen analysis

REFERENCES

Brit J Urol. 1999; 83: 283–284.
Cochrane Database Sys Rev. 2007 (2): CD004112.
Amer Fam Physician. 1999; 60: 137–152.
J Fam Pract. 1999; 48: 719–721.
J Urol. 1991; 145: 341–344.

19 ■ NEWBORN CIRCUMCISION WITH GOMCO CLAMP

INDICATIONS

- Cultural practice
- Parental desire for circumcision

CONTRAINDICATIONS

- Hypospadias or epispadias or megaurethra
- Ambiguous genitalia
- Short penile shaft (< 1 cm) or penile webbing
- Coagulopathy
- Myelomeningocele
- Imperforate anus
- Acute illness
- Extreme prematurity or age > 8 weeks

EQUIPMENT

- Infant restraint board
- Sucrose-coated pacifier
- 1% lidocaine
- 1-ml syringe with 30-gauge needle
- Povidone-iodine or chlorhexidine prep
- Sterile gloves
- Sterile fenestrated drape
- Sterile 2 × 2-inch gauze pads
- Three straight hemostats
- Gomco clamp with appropriately-sized bell (usually size 1.3)
- Sterile 1/2-inch petrolatum gauze
- 6-inch blunt probe
- No. 10 scalpel
- Scissors with one blunt tip

TECHNIQUE

- Restrain infant.
- Sterile prep and drape of penis and scrotum.
- Dorsal penile block:
  - Insert needle posteromedially about 0.5 cm at 2 o'clock and at 10 o'clock.
  - Inject 0.4 ml 1% lidocaine on each side.
- Sucrose-coated pacifier can also help diminish pain.
- Grasp foreskin with hemostats at 2 o'clock and at 10 o'clock and pull slight traction.
- Insert third hemostat or use blunt probe at 12 o'clock, tenting up foreskin; advance to coronal sulcus; open hemostat or use probe to sweep both directions to break up adhesions; avoid frenulum area (at 6 o'clock) (**Figure 19-1**).
- Lift grasping hemostats; advance lower blade of third hemostat at 12 o'clock until 1 cm from coronal sulcus; clamp third hemostat for 60 seconds, then remove (**Figure 19-2**).
- Cut foreskin along clamped line (**Figure 19-3**).

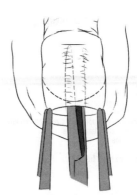

FIGURE 19-1. Clearing Adhesions Between Foreskin and Glans
Adapted from Pfenninger JL, Fowler GC, eds. *Procedures for Primary Care.* Philadelphia, PA: Elsevier; 2011: 1213, Figure 181-2.

A hemostat is used to break up adhesions under the foreskin.

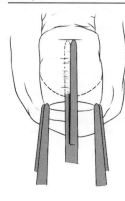

FIGURE 19-2. Creating a Dorsal Foreskin Crush

Adapted from Peleg D, Steiner A. The Gomco Circumcision: Common Problems and Solutions. *Amer Fam Physician.* 1998; 58(4): 894, Figure 4A.

A dorsal hemostat is applied with its tip 1 cm from the coronal sulcus to crush the dorsal foreskin.

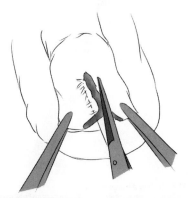

FIGURE 19-3. Creating a Dorsal Slit

Adapted from Peleg D, Steiner A. The Gomco Circumcision: Common Problems and Solutions. *Amer Fam Physician.* 1998; 58(4): 894, Figure 4A.

The foreskin is incised along the crushed line to create a dorsal slit.

- Retract foreskin behind glans and use gauze pads to free up any remaining adhesions.
- Place Gomco bell over glans (should barely cover complete glans).
- Clip dorsal slip edges together with a hemostat midway down dorsal slip (**Figure 19-4**).
  - Alternatively, a safety pin instead of a hemostat can be used to clip the dorsal slip edges together.
- Bring stem of bell and foreskin through the hole of Gomco clamp; use a hemostat to pull the foreskin symmetrically through the hole; release lower hemostat; elevate foreskin until the apex of dorsal slit is seen above the clamp (**Figure 19-5**).
  - If a safety pin is used, the pin can be pulled through the hole of the Gomco clamp to elevate the cut foreskin above the clamp.
- Secure bell to clamp and tighten screw completely where it touches the clamp.

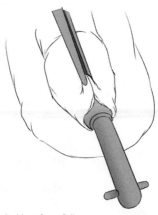

FIGURE 19-4. Applying a Gomco Bell
Adapted from Peleg D, Steiner A. The Gomco Circumcision: Common Problems and Solutions. *Amer Fam Physician.* 1998; 58(4): 894, Figure 4B.

Use a hemostat to reapproximate the dorsal slit around the Gomco bell.

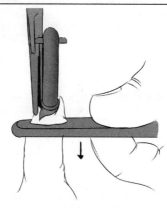

FIGURE 19-5. Elevating the Foreskin Through the Base Plate

Adapted from Peleg D, Steiner A. The Gomco Circumcision: Common Problems and Solutions. *Amer Fam Physician.* 1998; 58(4): 894, Figure 4D.

Elevate the stem of the Gomco bell and the foreskin through the base plate hole. Use a hemostat to pull the foreskin symmetrically through the hole until the apex of the dorsal slit is visualized.

- Use scalpel to cut foreskin circumferentially just above the baseplate (**Figure 19-6**).
  - Make sure that the cut edges are free of any tags of foreskin.
- Maintain the clamp in place for at least 5 minutes to prevent bleeding upon removal.
- Disassemble clamp and tease foreskin off bell using a gauze pad.
- Bleeding can usually be controlled with pressure +/- Surgicel.
- Wrap petrolatum gauze around glans and replace diaper.

POSTPROCEDURE CARE

- Remove petrolatum gauze in 24 hours.
- Reapply petrolatum jelly to glans with each diaper change.

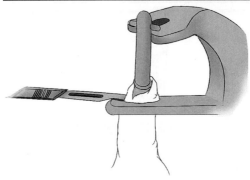

FIGURE 19-6. Excising the Foreskin
Adapted from Peleg D, Steiner A. The Gomco Circumcision: Common Problems and Solutions.
Amer Fam Physician. 1998; 58(4): 894, Figure 4F.

Excise the foreskin around the Gomco bell using a scalpel.

COMPLICATIONS

- Bleeding (0.1–1%)
- Infection (0.06–0.4%)
- Injury to glans or urethra (very rare)
- Meatal stenosis (very rare)
- Degloving injury of the penile shaft skin (especially if bell chosen is too large)
- Poor cosmetic result

CODING

54150   Circumcision, using clamp or other device; newborn

REFERENCES

Amer Fam Physician. 1995; 52: 511–518.
Amer Fam Physician. 1999; 58: 891–898.
Cochrane Database Syst Rev. 2004 (3): CD004217. *Urol Clin N Amer.* 2004; 31: 461–467.
Obstet Gynecol Surv. 2004; 59: 379–395.
Pfenninger JL, Fowler GL, eds. *Procedures for Primary Care.* Philadelphia, PA: Elsevier; 2011: 1211–1219.

SECTION VIII

GYNECOLOGIC PROCEDURES

20 ■ PAP SMEAR

- Cervical cancer screening
- Follow-up cervical dysplasia/cancer therapy

RELATIVE CONTRAINDICATIONS

- Active vaginitis, cervicitis, or pelvic inflammatory disease
- Active menstrual bleeding
- Severe anxiety about pelvic/speculum exams (may warrant procedural sedation)

EQUIPMENT

- Nonsterile gloves
- Warm speculum
- Water-soluble lubricant
- Cotton swabs
- Wooden or plastic spatula
- Cytobrush
- Microscope slides
- Fixative spray
- Alternative sampler: a "broom device"
- Alternative: media for liquid-based Pap smears (e.g., ThinPrep)

TECHNIQUE OF TRADITIONAL PAP SMEAR

- Patient in lithotomy position with feet in stirrups.
- Warm, lubricated speculum introduced and opened to visualize cervix.
- Using a large cotton swab, gently remove excess mucous from ectocervix.
- Place spatula onto ectocervix and gently rotate 360° (**Figure 20-1**).
- Insert Cytobrush into endocervical canal and rotate 90–180°; then withdraw (**Figure 20-2**).
  - Avoid this step in pregnancy.
- Sweep both sides of spatula across slide (**Figure 20-3**).

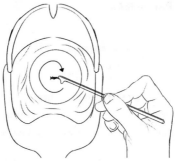

FIGURE 20-1. Sampling the Ectocervix With a Spatula
Adapted from Pfenninger JL, Fowler GC, eds. *Procedures for Primary Care*. Philadelphia, PA: Elsevier; 2011: 1028, Figure 151-3B.

Rotate spatula 360° to sample the ectocervix.

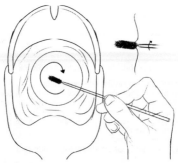

FIGURE 20-2. Sampling the Endocervical Canal With a Cytobrush
Adapted from Pfenninger JL, Fowler GC, eds. *Procedures for Primary Care*. Philadelphia, PA: Elsevier; 2011: 1028, Figure 151-3A.

Insert Cytobrush into endocervical canal and rotate 180°. Inset is the step in cross-section.

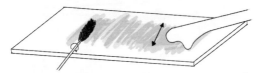

FIGURE 20-3. Smearing Sample on a Slide
Adapted from Pfenninger JL, Fowler GC, eds. *Procedures for Primary Care*. Philadelphia, PA: Elsevier; 2011: 1028, Figure 151-3C.

Smear both sides of the spatula and then roll the Cytobrush on a slide.

- Roll Cytobrush across the same slide (see **Figure 20-3**).
  - Alternative is to use a "broom device" (e.g., Papette or Cervex-Brush) and rotate 360° on the cervix five times (**Figure 20-4**).
  - Brush both sides of "broom" on a slide.
  - Avoid this device in pregnant patients.
- Spray slide with fixative (**Figure 20-5**).

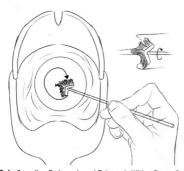

FIGURE 20-4. Sampling Endocervix and Ectocervix With a Broom Device
Adapted from Pfenninger JL, Fowler GC, eds. *Procedures for Primary Care*. Philadelphia, PA: Elsevier; 2011: 1028, Figure 151-3E.

Rotate "Broom" device 360° five times to sample endocervix and ectocervix. Inset is the step in cross-section.

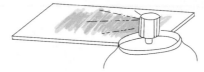

FIGURE 20-5. Preserving Specimen
Adapted from Pfenninger JL, Fowler GC, eds. *Procedures for Primary Care.* Philadelphia, PA: Elsevier; 2011: 1028, Figure 151-3D.

Spray fixative on smeared slides.

TECHNIQUE OF LIQUID-BASED PAP SMEAR

- Place spatula onto ectocervix and gently rotate 360° (see **Figure 20-1**).
- Insert Cytobrush into endocervical canal and rotate 90–180°; then withdraw (see **Figure 20-2**).
  - Avoid this device in pregnant patients.
- Swirl spatula in a vial of PreservCyt solution 10–20 revolutions (**Figure 20-6**).
- Aggressively scrape Cytobrush with spatula and spin Cytobrush in the same vial 10 revolutions; then cap vial (see **Figure 20-6**).

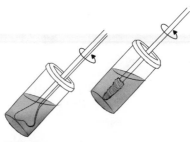

FIGURE 20-6. Liquid-Based Pap Testing
Adapted from Pfenninger JL, Fowler GC, eds. *Procedures for Primary Care.* Philadelphia, PA: Elsevier; 2011: 1028, Figures 151-4A and 151-4B.

Rotate spatula (A) and Cytobrush (B) each 10–20 revolutions within transport media for liquid-based Pap testing.

POSTPROCEDURE EVALUATION

- "Reflex" HPV DNA testing is available if cytologic abnormalities are detected with liquid-based Pap smears, but not with conventional Pap smears.
- All cytologic abnormalities should be assessed for whether colposcopy is indicated or HPV DNA testing is indicated.

COMPLICATIONS

- Vaginal spotting
- False negative Pap smears

CODING

88164	Obtaining and preparing a traditional screening Pap smear
88142	Obtaining and preparing a liquid-based screening Pap smear

REFERENCES

Gyn Onc. 2009; 112: 572–576.
J Clin Virology. 2009; 45 (S1): S3–S12.
Amer Fam Physician. 2009; 80: 147–155.
Pfenninger JL, Fowler GL, eds. *Procedures for Primary Care.* Philadelphia, PA: Elsevier; 2011: 1023–1032.

21 ■ ENDOMETRIAL BIOPSY

INDICATIONS

- Evaluation of abnormal vaginal bleeding
- Evaluate for a luteal phase defect (endometrial dating)
- Evaluation of atypical glandular cells of undetermined significance
- Evaluation of abnormal endometrial thickness seen by pelvic ultrasonography
- History of hereditary nonpolyposis colon cancer syndrome

CONTRAINDICATIONS

- Pregnancy
- Cervical stenosis
- Active vaginitis, cervicitis, or pelvic inflammatory disease
- Coagulopathy (relative)

EQUIPMENT

- Nonsterile gloves
- Sterile gloves
- Warm sterile speculum
- Water-soluble lubricant
- Cup of povidone-iodine
- Cotton balls
- Ring forceps
- Uterine sound
- Single-toothed tenaculum
- 20% benzocaine spray with long nozzle
- Plastic endometrial aspirator (e.g., Pipelle, Pipet Curet, or Endocell)
- Specimen jar with formalin
- Silver nitrate sticks

TECHNIQUE

- Patient in lithotomy position with feet in stirrups.
- Bimanual exam using non-sterile gloves to determine the size and orientation of uterus.
- Warm, lubricated speculum introduced and opened to visualize cervix.
- Change to sterile gloves.
- Have assistant spray cervix with 20% benzocaine.

- Dip cotton balls in povidone-iodine.
- Grasp cotton balls with ring forceps to prep cervix.
- Grasp anterior cervix with a single-toothed tenaculum.
- Sound uterus with gentle traction on tenaculum.
- Pass plastic endometrial aspirator into the uterus until the fundus is reached (**Figure 21-1**).
- Draw back the aspirator's internal piston (**Figure 21-2**); then rotate aspirator as it is moved back and forth from fundus toward cervix (**Figure 21-3**).
  - Withdraw plastic endometrial aspirator when the catheter fills with tissue.
  - Push piston back in to expel tissue into formalin (avoid contaminating aspirator) (**Figure 21-4**).
  - Repeat this step once.
- Remove tenaculum and use silver nitrate sticks to stop any oozing on cervix if bleeding is not stopped with gentle pressure using a cotton ball held in a ring forcep.
- Remove speculum.

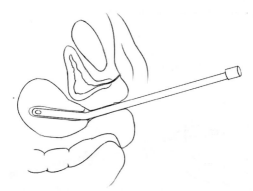

FIGURE 21-1. Insertion of Endometrial Aspirator

Adapted from Zuber TJ. Endometrial Biopsy. *Amer Fam Physician*, 2001; 63(6): 1133, Figure 1A.

The endometrial aspirator is inserted into the uterine cavity to the level of the fundus.

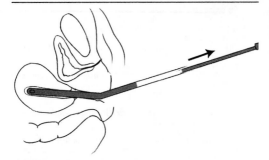

FIGURE 21-2. Withdrawal of Internal Piston
Adapted from Zuber TJ. Endometrial Biopsy. *Amer Fam Physician*, 2001; 63(6): 1133, Figure 1B.

Once inserted, the internal piston is fully withdrawn.

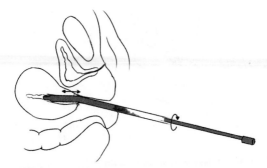

FIGURE 21-3. Endometrial Sampling
Adapted from Zuber TJ. Endometrial Biopsy. *Amer Fam Physician*, 2001; 63(6): 1133, Figure 1C.

Rotate the endometrial aspirator and simultaneously move the aspirator back and forth to sample the entire endometrial lining.

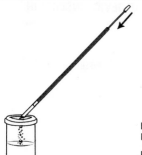

FIGURE 21-4. Sample Expelled Into a Formalin Jar

Push the piston forward to expel tissue into a formalin jar. Avoid touching the jar or formalin if the Pipelle will be used again.

POSTPROCEDURE CARE

- NSAIDs as needed for pelvic cramping.
- Avoid intercourse until bleeding has stopped.

COMPLICATIONS

- Uterine perforation
- Excessive uterine bleeding
- Infection (very rare)

CODING

58100	Endometrial biopsy, without cervical dilation, any method
59200	Insertion of cervical dilator (e.g., mechanical dilators or laminaria)

REFERENCES

Amer Fam Physician. 2001; 63: 1131–1135.
Obstet Gynecol Survey. 2009; 64: 249–257.
Prim Care Clin N Amer. 1997; 24: 303.
Med Sci Monitor. 2004; 10: CR271–MR274.

22 ■ INTRAUTERINE DEVICE INSERTION AND REMOVAL

INDICATIONS

- Contraception
- Endometriosis (Mirena)
- Dysmenorrhea (Mirena)
- Menorrhagia (Mirena)

CONTRAINDICATIONS

- Uterine cavity malformations
- Pregnancy
- Vaginal bleeding of unclear etiology
- Recent STD, septic abortion, or postpartum endometritis
- Suspected uterine/cervical malignancy
- History of ectopic pregnancy
- History of pelvic inflammatory disease since last pregnancy
- Gestational trophoblastic disease
- Genital actinomycosis
- Ovarian cancer
- Liver cancer
- Current or history of breast cancer (Mirena)
- HIV-positive patients
- Multiple current sexual partners (relative)
- Active viral hepatitis or advanced cirrhosis (Mirena)
- Complex migraines (Mirena)
- Active venous thromboembolism (Mirena)
- Allergy to copper (ParaGard T380A)
- Wilson's disease (ParaGard T380A)

EQUIPMENT

- Intrauterine device (Mirena or Paragard)
- Warm speculum
- Cup of povidone-iodine
- Cotton balls
- Ring forceps
- Single-toothed tenaculum
- Uterine sound
- Sterile and nonsterile gloves
- Long suture scissors

TECHNIQUE FOR PARAGARD T380A INSERTION

- Patient in dorsal lithotomy position with feet in stirrups.
- Confirm a negative Pap smear.
- Confirm a negative GC/chlamydia test within the last month.
- Confirm a negative pregnancy test.
- Perform a bimanual exam to assess uterine size and position.
- Introduce speculum to visualize cervix; then change to sterile gloves.
- Prep cervix with povidone-iodine.
- Attempt to sound uterus if bimanual exam indicates that the uterus is not significantly anteverted or retroverted.
- If unable to easily enter through internal os:
  * Place tenaculum on anterior lip of cervix.
  * Sound the uterus with gentle traction of tenaculum (adequate uterine depth is 6–9 cm).
- Adjust position of the blue flange to equal the distance of the measured uterine size.
- Fold the arms of the IUD parallel to the body and push them into the IUD insertion unit (**Figure 22-1**).
- Insert the IUD tube through the cervix until blue flange is at the cervix (**Figure 22-2**).

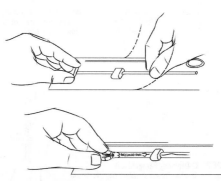

FIGURE 22-1. Preparing Paragard IUD
Adapted from Insertion Process. ParaGard Web site. http://www.paraguard.com/hcp/insertion-training: Steps 1 and 2. Accessed September 28, 2010.

Within the package, insert the arms of the IUD into the insertion tube.

- Place the inserter rod securely on the IUD; then retract clear inserter tube, keeping the inserter rod in place to deploy IUD **(Figure 22-3)**.
- Keep insertion tube in place as insertion rod is removed.
- Remove insertion tube and tenaculum.
- Trim IUD strings to length of 3 cm.

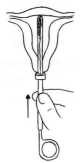

FIGURE 22-2. Insertion of Paragard IUD
Adapted from Insertion Process. ParaGard Web site. http://www.paraguard.com/hcp/insertion-training: Step 3. Accessed September 28, 2010.

The flange is adjusted based on the uterine depth as determined by a uterine sound. The Paragard IUD is inserted until the flange touches the cervix.

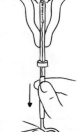

FIGURE 22-3. Deploying Paragard IUD
Adapted from Insertion Process. ParaGard Web site. http://www.paraguard.com/hcp/insertion-training: Step 4. Accessed September 28, 2010.

A probe is inserted through the insertion tube until it touches the IUD. The insertion tube is then retracted, keeping the probe stationary to deploy the IUD.

TECHNIQUE FOR MIRENA IUD INSERTION

- Follow steps above through uterine sounding.
- Release threads of Mirena.
- Assure that slider is pushed away from you (**Figure 22-4**).
- Pull strings to draw arms fully within the insertion tube (**Figure 22-5**).
- Place strings within groove on handle.
- Adjust flange to equal the distance of the measured uterine size.
- Insert IUD while holding the slider firmly; advance until flange is 1.5 cm from cervix (**Figure 22-6**).
- Hold inserter steady while slider is pulled back to a black mark on handle (**Figure 22-7**).
- Push inserter forward until flange touches cervix.
- Hold inserter steady and pull slider all the way back; this automatically releases strings (**Figure 22-8**).
- Remove inserter.
- Trim strings to 3 cm length.

POSTPROCEDURE CARE

- Check for presence of IUD strings after each menstrual period.
- Replacement: ParaGard = 10 yrs; Mirena = 5 yrs.

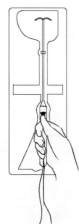

FIGURE 22-4. Preparing Mirena IUD
Adapted from Mirena [package insert]. Bayer HealthCare Pharmaceuticals Inc. Wayne, NJ; October 2009. http://berlex.bayerhealthcare.com/html/products/pi/Mirena_PI.pdf: 3, Figure 1B. Accessed September 28, 2010.

Align the IUD arms with the slider in the farthest position.

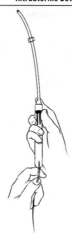

FIGURE 22-5. Loading Mirena IUD
Adapted from Mirena [package insert]. Bayer HealthCare Pharmaceuticals Inc. Wayne, NJ; October 2009. http://berlex.bayerhealthcare.com/html/products/pi/Mirena_PI.pdf: 3, Figure 2A. Accessed September 28, 2010.

Holding the slider in the furthest position, pull the threads to load the Mirena in the insertion tube.

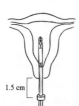

1.5 cm

FIGURE 22-6. Insertion of Mirena IUD
Adapted from Mirena [package insert]. Bayer HealthCare Pharmaceuticals Inc. Wayne, NJ; October 2009. http://berlex.bayer healthcare.com/html/products/pi/Mirena_PI.pdf: 4, Figure 5. Accessed September 28, 2010.

The flange is adjusted based on the uterine depth as determined by a uterine sound. While holding the slider in the furthest position, insert the IUD into the uterine cavity until the flange is 1.5 cm from the cervical os.

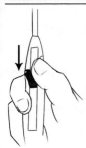

FIGURE 22-7. Deploying Mirena IUD
Adapted from Mirena [package insert]. Bayer HealthCare Pharmaceuticals Inc. Wayne, NJ; October 2009. http://ber-lex.bayerhealthcare.com/html/products/pi/Mirena_PI.pdf: 4, Figure 6A. Accessed September 28, 2010.

Pull slider back to the black mark to release the arms of the Mirena IUD. Then advance the insertion tube until the flange touches the cervix.

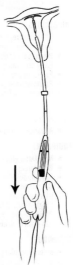

FIGURE 22-8. Releasing IUD
Adapted from Mirena [package insert]. Bayer HealthCare Pharmaceuticals Inc. Wayne, NJ; October 2009. http://berlex.bayerhealthcare.com/html/products/pi/Mirena_PI.pdf: 4, Figure 8. Accessed September 28, 2010.

Pull the slider all the way back, which releases the threads. Then withdraw the insertion tube completely out of the cervix.

COMPLICATIONS

- Uterine perforation (0.1%)
- Irregular vaginal bleeding (especially in first 3 months)
- Expulsion of IUD
- Migration of IUD
- Ectopic pregnancy
- Pelvic inflammatory disease (especially in first three weeks post-insertion)
- Vasovagal reaction (on insertion)
- Actinomyces infection (usually asymptomatic)
- Mirena-specific adverse reactions
  - Amenorrhea; acne; depression; weight gain; decreased libido; headache

CODING

58300   Intrauterine device insertion

INTRAUTERINE DEVICE REMOVAL

INDICATIONS

- IUD needs replacement
- Request for removal
- Pelvic pain or dyspareunia
- Early pregnancy
- Pelvic inflammatory disease
- Pelvic actinomycosis
- IUD contraindication develops
- Need for excisional procedure of cervix

CONTRAINDICATIONS

- Advanced pregnancy

EQUIPMENT

- Nonsterile gloves
- Ring forceps
- Speculum
- Cytobrush
- Uterine sound
- Single-toothed tenaculum
- Povidone-iodine swabs
- IUD hook or double IUD extractor

TECHNIQUE

- Insert speculum.

- When IUD strings visible, grasp them with ring forceps and pull gentle traction until body of IUD visible.
- Grasp body of IUD with ring forceps and pull out.
- If IUD strings are not visible:
  - Insert Cytobrush to the full depth; rotate several times; withdraw while rotating.
  - If strings visible, remove IUD as above.
  - If unsuccessful, obtain a pelvic ultrasound to assure IUD is within the uterus.
  - If IUD is in the uterine cavity, prep cervix with povidone-iodine.
  - Apply tenaculum to anterior lip of cervix.
  - Sound uterus.
  - Insert double IUD extractor and try to snag IUD or its strings and pull it out.
  - If unsuccessful, refer for hysteroscopic removal.

POSTPROCEDURE CARE

- Alternative contraception if needed

COMPLICATIONS

- Uterine perforation or infection if double IUD extractor or IUD hook used

CODING

58301   Intrauterine device removal

REFERENCES

Amer Fam Physician. 2005; 71: 95–102.
Mirena [package insert]. Montville, NJ: Berlex Laboratories; 2003. ParaGard [package insert]. Tonawanda, NY: FEI Products; 2003.
Obstet Clin N Amer. 2000; 27: 723–740.
ACOG Practice Bulletin. 2005; 59: 1–10.
Obstet Clin N Amer. 2000; 27: 723–740.
J Fam Practice. 2006; 55: 726–729.

SECTION IX

HEMATOLOGY/ONCOLOGY PROCEDURES

23 ■ BONE MARROW ASPIRATION AND BIOPSY

INDICATIONS

- Evaluation of unexplained anemia
- Evaluation of unexplained thrombocytopenia
- Evaluation of unexplained pancytopenia
- Evaluation of unexplained leukopenia
- Diagnosis of multiple myeloma
- Workup of fever of unknown origin in immunocompromised patients
- Diagnosis and staging of lymphoma and leukemia
- Workup for bone marrow transplantation
- Workup of unexplained splenomegaly
- Workup of possible lysosomal storage disease
- Workup of primary amyloidosis
- Staging for small cell tumors of childhood
- Samples for chromosomal analysis

CONTRAINDICATIONS

- Uncooperative patient
- Skin or bone infection at intended biopsy site
- Previous radiation therapy at intended biopsy site (relative)
- Severe osteoporosis (relative)
- Myeloma or severe osteoporosis is an absolute contraindication for sternal bone marrow sampling

EQUIPMENT

- Prepackaged Jamshidi bone marrow aspiration and biopsy kit
  - 1% lidocaine
  - Sterile prep: chlorhexidine or povidone-iodine swabs
  - Sterile 4 × 4-inch gauze pack
  - 5-ml and 20-ml syringes
  - 18-gauge, 22-gauge, and 25-gauge needles
  - Sterile Band-aid
  - Glass slides (10)
- Green-top (sodium heparin) tube if flow cytometry, cytogenetics or molecular gene rearrangement studies needed

- Culture bottles if infectious etiology is to be ruled out
  - May include special bottles for acid-fast bacilli, fungus, or bacterial cultures (anaerobic and aerobic bottles)
- Jar of formalin

BIOPSY SITES

- Posterior superior iliac spine (**Figure 23-1**)
  - Most common site in adults or children older than 1 year of age
  - Can obtain aspirate and core biopsy
- Anterior superior iliac spine
  - Alternative site for adults and older children
  - Can obtain aspirate and core biopsy
- Sternum
  - Bone marrow aspirate only in age > 12 years (not for core biopsies)
- Anterior tibia
  - Premature or term infants and toddlers < 18 months
  - Can obtain aspirate and core biopsy

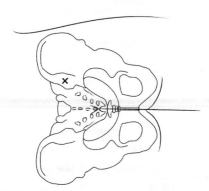

FIGURE 23-1. Landmarks For Posterior Superior Iliac Spine Bone Marrow Biopsy
Adapted from Knowles S, Hoffbrand AV. Bone Marrow Aspiration and Trephine Biopsy. *Brit Med J.* 1980; 281(6234): 204, Figure 1.

The landmarks for a posterior superior iliac spine (PSIS) bone marrow biopsy are the PSIS and the top of the gluteal cleft. If the PSIS is not palpable, the PSIS is approximately 3–4 finger-breadths superior to and lateral to the top of the gluteal cleft.

TECHNIQUE FOR POSTERIOR SUPERIOR ILIAC SPINE BONE MARROW ASPIRATE

- Informed consent.
- Perform a "time out" procedure to confirm correct patient, site, and procedure.
- Consider procedural sedation for patients who have severe anxiety or a low pain threshold.
  - Can use hydromorphone 1–2 mg PO and lorazepam 1–2 mg PO one hour before procedure.
- Positioning:
  - Prone (preferred position)
  - Lateral decubitus position with knees flexed (alternative position)
- Identify posterior superior iliac spine (see **Figure 23-1**).
  - Approximately 3–4 finger-breadths superior to and lateral to top of the gluteal cleft
- Sterile prep and drape of posterior iliac crest area.
- Anesthetize skin and periosteum with 1% lidocaine.
  - Use at least 5 ml lidocaine and anesthetize a 1-cm area of periosteum
- Insert marrow aspiration needle perpendicular to bone.
- Drive needle into bone with rotating motion.
- Stop when one feels a loss of resistance signifying penetration through cortex (**Figure 23-2**).
  - The needle should not wobble in the bone.

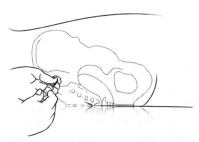

FIGURE 23-2. Introducing a Bone Marrow Aspirate Needle

A bone marrow aspirate needle is introduced through the bony cortex of the posterior superior iliac spine. At this point, the needle should be stationary and not wobble back and forth.

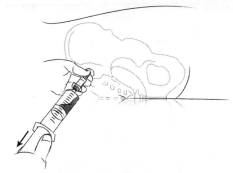

FIGURE 23-3. Obtaining a Bone Marrow Aspirate

A 20-ml syringe is attached to the bone marrow aspirate needle and the plunger is withdrawn to aspirate a sample of bone marrow.

- Remove stylet and firmly attach a 20-ml syringe to needle.
- Quickly pull up on plunger and aspirate 5 ml of marrow for routine studies (**Figure 23-3**).
  - Additional marrow volume may be required if additional studies are needed.
- Give syringe to a hematology technician to prepare slides.
  - Many bony spicules represents a good bone marrow sample.

TECHNIQUE FOR POSTERIOR SUPERIOR ILIAC SPINE BONE MARROW CORE BIOPSY

- Use a Jamshidi biopsy needle.
- Advance needle perpendicular to bone in rotating manner (**Figure 23-4**).
- Once cortex is penetrated, unscrew cap and remove stylet (**Figure 23-5**).
- Advance needle an additional 1.5 cm with wide sweeping rotating twists (**Figure 23-6**).
- Turn needle 360° three times in each direction; rock needle between each turn.
- Slowly withdraw needle while rotating needle clockwise and counterclockwise.
- Push bone marrow core specimen out of needle using a metal probe (**Figure 23-7**).

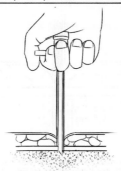

FIGURE 23-4. Advancing Jamshidi Needle Through Bony Cortex
Adapted from Choby BA. Bone Marrow Aspiration and Biopsy. In: Pfenninger JL, Fowler GC, eds. *Procedures for Primary Care*. Philadelphia, PA: Elsevier, Inc., 2011: 1406, Figure 205-6A.

A Jamshidi needle is advanced with a rotating motion through the bony cortex of the posterior superior iliac spine. Once through the cortex, it should be stationary and not wobble back and forth.

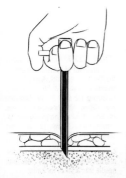

FIGURE 23-5. Removing Stylet From Jamshidi Needle

Once the Jamshidi needle is inserted through the bony cortex, the cap and inner stylet are removed.

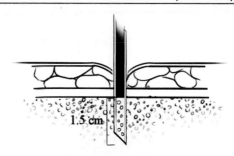

FIGURE 23-6. Advancing Jamshidi Needle Into Bone Marrow
Adapted from Choby BA. Bone Marrow Aspiration and Biopsy. In: Pfenninger JL, Fowler GC, eds. *Procedures for Primary Care.* Philadelphia, PA: Elsevier, Inc., 2011: 1406, Figure 205-6B.

The Jamshidi needle is advanced an additional 1–1.5 cm with a twisting motion. A cylindrical core of bone marrow fills the hollow needle during this part of the procedure.

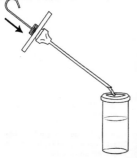

FIGURE 23-7. Pushing Biopsy Specimen Out of Jamshidi Needle
Adapted from Riley RS, Rosenblum D, Forsythe R, et al. *An Illustrated Guide to Performing the Bone Marrow Aspiration and Biopsy.* http://www.pathology.vcu.edu/education/PathLab/pages/hematopath/bm.html: Figure 12. Accessed September 28, 2010.

A probe is used to push the bone marrow core out of the Jamshidi needle into a jar of formalin.

- Touch preparation (roll core biopsy on slide) if marrow not aspirable.
- Place bone marrow core biopsy into formalin.
- Band-aid and ice pack to biopsy site.

BONE MARROW ASPIRATE OPTIONAL STUDIES

- Bone marrow aspirate in sodium heparin (green-top) tube
  - Flow cytometry for leukemia/lymphoma/myeloma
  - Cytogenetic analysis
  - Molecular cytogenetics (by FISH analysis)
  - Gene rearrangement studies by polymerase chain reaction

COMPLICATIONS

- Infection at biopsy site (extremely rare)
- Bleeding at biopsy site (extremely rare)
- Local pain (usually transient in nature)
- Cardiac tamponade (in sternal biopsies, rare)
- Serious adverse events occur in about 1 in 2000 procedures

CODING

38220   Bone marrow aspiration

38221   Bone marrow biopsy

REFERENCES

J. Clinical Pathology. 2001; 54: 657–663.
J Clin Pathol. 2001; 54: 773–742.
Hematology Oncology Clin. N. America. 1988; 2: 513.
Southern Medical J. 1999; 92: 477.
British J. Haematology. 2003; 121: 821.
J Clin Lab Analysis. 2004; 18: 70–90.
NEJM. 2009; 361: e28.
Pfenninger JL, Fowler GC, eds. *Procedures for Primary Care.* Philadelphia, PA: Elsevier; 2011: 1404–1408.

SECTION X

NEUROLOGY PROCEDURES

24 ■ LUMBAR PUNCTURE

- **Diagnostic Lumbar Puncture**
  - Meningitis (bacterial, fungal, tuberculous, carcinomatosis, lymphomatosis, or aseptic)
  - Early subarachnoid hemorrhage
  - Pseudotumor cerebri
  - Multiple sclerosis
  - Guillain-Barré syndrome
  - Possible lupus cerebritis, CNS vasculitis, or acute demyelinating disorders
- **Therapeutic Lumbar Puncture**
  - Spinal anesthesia
  - Treatment of pseudotumor cerebri
  - Adjunctive therapy for cryptococcal meningitis
  - Intrathecal injection of chemotherapy or antimicrobials
  - Injection of contrast media for myelography or cisternography

CONTRAINDICATIONS

- Uncooperative patient
- Infection at the insertion site
- Elevated intracranial pressure
- Intracranial mass
- Obstructive hydrocephalus
- Thrombocytopenia (platelets < 50,000)
- Coagulopathy (INR > 1.4 or PTT > 1.5 × upper limit of normal)
- CT findings that are absolute contraindications: midline shift; loss of suprachiasmatic and basilar cisterns; posterior fossa mass; loss of superior cerebellar cistern; or loss of quadrigeminal plate cistern

EQUIPMENT

- Face mask
- Sterile gloves and gown
- 1% lidocaine solution
- 22-gauge and 25-gauge needles

- 5-ml labeled syringe for local anesthesia
- Povidone-iodine prep
- Sterile drape
- Spinal needle with stylet
  - 22-gauge, 3.5-inch spinal needle for adults
  - 22-gauge, 2.5-inch spinal needle for children
  - 22-gauge, 1.5-inch spinal needle for infants and newborns
- Manometer with three-way stopcock
- Four labeled sterile specimen containers
- Sterile bandage

TECHNIQUE

- Position:
  - Lateral decubitus (keep shoulders and hips aligned)
  - Sitting
- Prep back with povidone-iodine and sterile drape.
- Anesthetize skin at either the L_{3-4} or L_{2-3} interspace.
  - The top of the iliac crests is at the L_4 vertebral body (**Figure 24-1**).
  - Ultrasound can identify the interspace if landmarks are difficult to palpate secondary to obese body habitus.
- Introduce spinal needle in the interspace angled 15° cephalad toward umbilicus (see **Figure 24-1**).
- Advance needle with the bevel facing toward the patients side until a "pop" is felt.
  - Typical insertion depth in newborns is ~1.5 cm (0.6 inches).
  - Typical insertion depth in infants is 1.5–2 cm (0.6–0.8 inches).
  - Typical insertion depth in young children is 3–4 cm (1.2–1.6 inches).
  - Typical insertion depth in older or obese children is 4–5 cm (1.6–2 inches).
  - Typical insertion depth in average-sized adults is 50–75% the length of the needle.
  - Typical insertion depth in obese adults is 75–90% the length of the needle.
- Withdraw stylet and check for fluid return (**Figure 24-2**).
- If no fluid return, consider the depth of insertion, alignment with landmarks, and needle angle in the sagittal plane.
- Attach end of stopcock with manometer to read the opening pressure (**Figure 24-3**).
  - Opening pressure can only be checked in lateral decubitus position.
- Collect 1–2 ml CSF in each of the four labeled sterile tubes (**Figure 24-4**).
- Replace stylet and withdraw the spinal needle.
- Clean off povidone-iodine prep solution.
- Apply a sterile Band-aid over the puncture site.

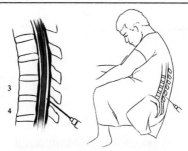

FIGURE 24-1. Insertion of Spinal Needle In the L3-4 Interspace

The spinal needle is introduced parallel to the floor at a 15° angle cephalad toward the umbilicus. The iliac crests have been outlined as have the posterior spinous processes. The L4 vertebrae is aligned with the top of the iliac crest.

FIGURE 24-2. The Stylet Is Removed From the Spinal Needle

The spinal needle is introduced until a "pop," or loss of resistance, is appreciated. Then the stylet is removed to check for return of cerebrospinal fluid.

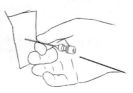

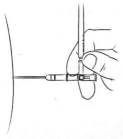

FIGURE 24-3. Attaching a Manometer To the Spinal Needle

A manometer is attached to the hub of the spinal needle with the patient in the lateral decubitus position to check the opening pressure.

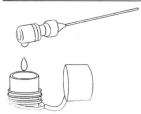

FIGURE 24-4. Collecting CSF In Sterile Collection Tubes

CSF is collected in sterile collection tubes. The stylet is then replaced within the spinal needle prior to withdrawing the needle from the skin.

CEREBROSPINAL FLUID STUDIES (TABLE 24-1)

- Routine Studies
  - Cell count with differential; glucose; protein; culture and gram stain
- Optional studies
  - Infectious studies: VDRL; cocci titer; AFB RNA by PCR; India ink; cryptococcal antigen; adenosine deaminase level; lactate; and encephalitis panel
  - Noninfectious: multiple sclerosis panel; cytology; angiotensin converting enzyme (ACE) levels (neurosarcoidosis)

WHEN TO OBTAIN A CT SCAN OF THE HEAD PRIOR TO A LUMBAR PUNCTURE

- **Needed for the presence of any of these clinical risk factors that suggest increased ICP**
  - Altered mental status (LR 2.2)
  - Focal deficit (LR 4.3)
  - Papilledema (LR 11)
- **Not needed if all of the following are absent (LR 0.1)**
  - Age ≥ 60
  - Immunocompromised state
  - History of CNS disease
  - Seizure in last week
  - Abnormal level of consciousness
  - Inability to answer two questions correctly
  - Inability to follow two consecutive commands correctly
  - Gaze palsy
  - Abnormal visual fields
  - Facial palsy
  - Arm (or pronator) drift
  - Leg weakness
  - Abnormal speech or language

TABLE 24-1. Normal CSF Values in Adults

Opening pressure 60–200 mm H$_2$0	Protein 15–45 mg/dl	Gram stain: no organisms
Glucose ≥ 60% serum glucose	WBC ≤ 5/mm^3 (subtract 1 WBC per 700 RBC in CSF)	

PREDICTORS OF BACTERIAL MENINGITIS

- CSF WBC ≥ 500/μl (likelihood ratio = 15)
- CSF glucose/blood glucose ≤ 0.4 (likelihood ratio = 18)
- CSF lactate ≥ 31.5 mg/dl (likelihood ratio = 21)

COMPLICATIONS

- **Major**
  - Brain herniation (if elevated intracranial pressure)
  - Epidural hematoma
  - Epidural abscess or diskitis
  - Seizure
- **Minor**
  - Spinal headache
  - Local back pain
  - Lower extremity paresthesias

CODING

62270	Lumbar puncture, diagnostic
62272	Lumbar puncture, therapeutic for drainage of spinal fluid
76942	Ultrasound-guidance

REFERENCES

JAMA. 2006; 296: 2012–2022.
NEJM. 2006; 355: e12.
Roberts, JR, Hedges JR, eds. *Clinical Procedures in Emergency Medicine*. 5th ed. Philadelphia, PA: Saunders; 2009: 1107–1127.

SECTION XI

ORTHOPEDICS PROCEDURES

25 ■ SPLINTING AND CASTING OF THE EXTREMITIES

INDICATIONS FOR SPLINTING

- Any condition that requires immobilization
- Severe sprains
- Tenosynovitis
- Reduced joint dislocations
- Acute fractures or suspected fractures with a negative x-ray (e.g., Scaphoid or Supracondylar fractures)
- Complex lacerations across joints

INDICATIONS FOR CASTING

- Need for prolonged immobilization
  - Extremity fractures
  - Total-contact cast for nonhealing diabetic foot ulcers
  - Congenital deformities (e.g., talipes equinovarus or clubfoot deformities)

CONTRAINDICATIONS

- Unstable fractures
- Open fractures
- Fracture associated with acute infection (cast)

EQUIPMENT

- Stockinette
- Towels or absorbent pads
- Webril (padding)
- Elastic wrap (e.g., Ace wrap or Bias roll)
- Plaster or fiberglass casting material
- Bandage scissors
- Nonsterile gloves
- Basin of clean, lukewarm water
- Adhesive tape or clips (for splints)
- Towels or chux

BASIC TECHNIQUE FOR SPLINTING EXTREMITIES

- Cut stockinette 10 cm longer than intended splint length.
- Apply stockinette with each side extending 5 cm beyond splint site
  (**Figure 25-1**).
  - Cut hole for thumb.
- Keep the joints in the position of function.
  - Hand in the "wineglass position" if fingers will **not** be immobilized
    (**Figure 25-2**)
  - Keep metacarpal joints at 90° and fingers extended if **fingers
    immobilized**
  - Ankle kept at 90°
  - Elbow at 90°

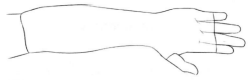

FIGURE 25-1. Stockinette Application

Stockinette should extend about 5 cm beyond each end of the intended splint
site.

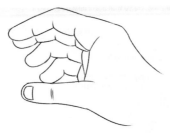

FIGURE 25-2. Position of Function of the Hand

Functional position of the hand is the "wineglass position" if fingers will **not**
be immobilized.

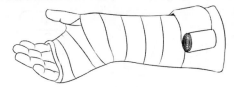

FIGURE 25-3. Wrap Cast Padding (Webril)

Adapted from Roberts JR, Hedges JR, eds. *Clinical Procedures in Emergency Medicine*. 5th ed. Philadelphia, PA: Saunders; 2009: 912 Figure 50-5B.

Wrap cast padding (Webril) to extend 2–3 cm beyond expected splint edges.

- Apply three layers of Webril to extend 2–3 cm beyond splint edges (**Figure 25-3**); apply extra padding on pressure points.
- Submerge the fiberglass or plaster (until bubbling stops); do not oversoak.
- Squeeze off excess water.
- Use towels or absorbent pads to protect against spillage onto clothing.
  - Plaster that spills onto clothing washes off; fiberglass that touches clothing will ruin it.
- Apply splint smoothly; fold back stockinette/Webril (**Figure 25-4**).
  - If fingers are **not** immobilized, the splint should end at the distal palmar crease.
  - Short arm or short leg splints should not interfere with the full motion of the knee or elbow.
  - Wrap a single layer of Webril around fiberglass so the elastic wrap does not stick to it.

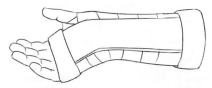

FIGURE 25-4. Applying Cast Material For Splinting

Adapted from Roberts JR, Hedges JR, eds. *Clinical Procedures in Emergency Medicine*. 5th ed. Philadelphia, PA: Saunders; 2009: 912 Figure 50-5C.

Apply moistened cast material and fold back stockinette and Webril over cast material.

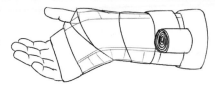

FIGURE 25-5. Wrapping Elastic Wrap Over Cast Material For Splinting
Adapted from Roberts JR, Hedges JR, eds. *Clinical Procedures in Emergency Medicine.* 5th ed.
Philadelphia, PA: Saunders; 2009: 912 Figure 50-5D.

Wrap elastic wrap over cast material to secure it in place. Secure elastic wrap
with clips and/or tape.

- Secure the splint with elastic wrap (**Figure 25-5**).
- Mold the splint with palms, not fingers, to conform to extremity (**Figure 25-9**).
- Perform a FACTS check: Function; Arterial pulse; Capillary refill; Temperature (of skin); Sensation.

BASIC TECHNIQUE FOR CASTING EXTREMITIES

- Repeat all the initial steps described in splinting section: Apply stockinette with joints in the position of function; apply Webril; submerge plaster or fiberglass; squeeze off excess water.
- Wrap casting material circumferentially overlapping the previous layer by 50% (**Figure 25-6**).
  - If fingers are **not** immobilized, the cast should end at the distal palmar crease.
  - Short arm or short leg casts should not interfere with the full motion of the knee or elbow.
- Cast must not be loose, but avoid excessive tension as material is rolled onto arm.
- After first layer of cast material applied, fold back stockinette and Webril padding (**Figure 25-7**).
- Apply a final layer of cast material over the stockinette and Webril (**Figure 25-8**).
- Mold the cast using your palms with the extremity in a position of function (see **Figure 25-9**).

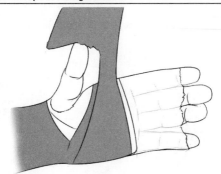

FIGURE 25-6. Application of Cast Material Over Webril For Casting

Application of cast material over Webril. The fiberglass material is cut at the level of the thumb and the free edges are folded underneath to develop a smooth edge around the thumb.

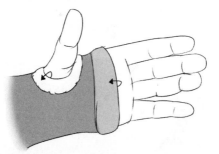

FIGURE 25-7. Folding Webril and Stockinette Over Cast Material

Folding Webril and stockinette over cast material at the thumb and the proximal and distal edges of the cast.

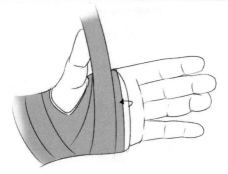

FIGURE 25-8. Rolling Cast Material Over the Webril and Stockinette

The cast material is rolled over the webril and stockinette that was folded back at the edges of the cast.

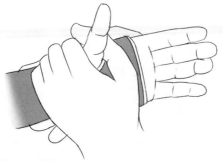

FIGURE 25-9. Molding the Cast Into the Proper Position

The palms of the hands are used to mold the cast into the proper position.

ARM SPLINTS

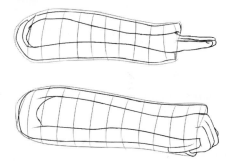

FIGURE 25-10. Sugar Tong Splint

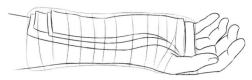

FIGURE 25-11. Volar Short Arm Splint

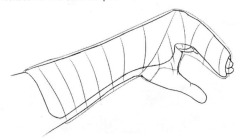

FIGURE 25-12. Ulnar Gutter Splint

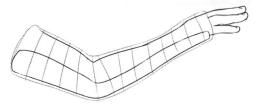

FIGURE 25-13. Posterior Long Arm Splint

ARM CASTS

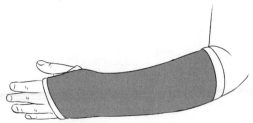

FIGURE 25-14. Short Arm Cast

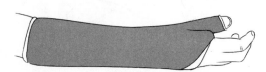

FIGURE 25-15. Thumb Spica Cast

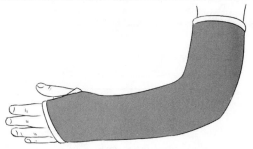

FIGURE 25-16. Long Arm Cast

LEG SPLINTS

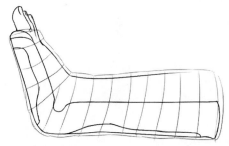

FIGURE 25-17. Posterior Leg Splint

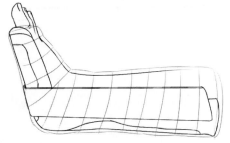

FIGURE 25-18. Posterior Leg and Stirrup Splints

LEG CASTS

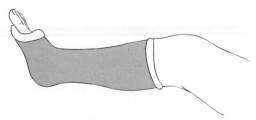

FIGURE 25-19. Short Leg Cast

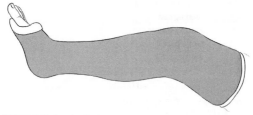

FIGURE 25-20. Long Leg Cast

POSTPROCEDURE CARE

- Keep splints and casts clean and dry.
- Never insert anything under the splint or cast material.
- Return for any fever, increased extremity pain, numbness, paresthesias, burning, discoloration of the fingers, or any drainage or bad odors emanating from the splint/cast.

COMPLICATIONS

- Compartment syndrome
- Extremity ischemia
- Heat injury to skin
- Pressure sores and skin injury
- Infection
- Dermatitis
- Neurologic injury

CODING

29065	Long arm cast
29075	Short arm cast
29049	Long arm splint (shoulder to hand)
29125	Short arm splint
29130	Finger splint
29345	Long leg cast

29355	Long leg walking cast
29405	Short leg cast
29425	Short leg walking cast
29505	Long leg splint
29515	Short leg splint

REFERENCES

Amer Fam Physician. 2009; 80: 491–499.
Amer Fam Physician. 2009; 79: 16–24.
Emer Med Clin N Amer. 2000; 18: 67–84.
Roberts JR, Hedges JR, eds. *Clinical Procedures in Emergency Medicine,* 5th ed. Philadelphia, PA: Saunders; 2009: page 912.

26 ■ ARTHROCENTESIS

INDICATIONS FOR DIAGNOSTIC ARTHROCENTESIS

- Evaluate for septic arthritis
- Evaluate for crystal-induced arthritis
- Differentiate between inflammatory and non-inflammatory arthritis
- Any persistent unexplained monoarthritis

INDICATIONS FOR THERAPEUTIC ARTHROCENTESIS

- Intra-articular injection of steroids, local anesthetic, or hyaluronic acid derivatives
- Drainage of large symptomatic joint effusions or hemarthroses

ABSOLUTE CONTRAINDICATIONS

- Skin infection at the site of needle insertion
- Allergy to injected medications
- Unstable joint

RELATIVE CONTRAINDICATIONS

- Coagulopathy
- Thrombocytopenia (platelets < 50,000)
- Aspiration of a prosthetic joint
- Bacteremia

EQUIPMENT

- Chlorhexidine or povidone-iodine swabs
- Sterile drape
- Absorbent underpads (e.g., Chux)
- Sterile gloves
- 18-gauge, 20-gauge, and 27-gauge needles, 1 1/2 inches
- 5-ml syringe for local anesthesia
- 1% lidocaine or Ethyl chloride spray
- 20–60-ml syringe for aspiration
- Hemostat
- Aerobic and anaerobic culture bottles for bedside inoculation

- EDTA purple-top tube (for cell count with differential)
- Red-top tube (for crystal analysis and gram stain)
- Sterile syringe cap
- Sterile bandage

TECHNIQUE FOR KNEE ARTHROCENTESIS

- Position: supine on bed with the rolled towel under knee for 15° flexion (large effusions).
  - Knee extended (for small effusions)
- Sterile prep and drape of knee.
- Anesthetize the skin and subcutaneous tissues at the insertion site with lidocaine or Ethyl chloride spray.
- Apply gentle pressure on contralateral side of knee to push joint fluid toward insertion site.
- Lateral approach:
  - Insertion site is 1 cm superior and 1 cm lateral to the superolateral edge of patella.
  - Introduce an 18-gauge needle at a 45° angle to the axis of the femur and parallel to the bed under patella with constant negative pressure (**Figure 26-1**).

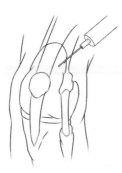

FIGURE 26-1. Knee Arthrocentesis

Adapted from Zuber TJ. Knee Joint Aspiration and Injection. *Amer Fam Physician.* 2002; 66(8): 1499, Figure 1.

Insert the needle 1 cm above and 1 cm lateral to the superior lateral aspect of the patella. The needle is introduced underneath the patella at a 45° angle.

- Medial approach:
  - Insertion site is in midportion of patella just beneath the patella.
  - Introduce an 18-gauge needle horizontal to the bed into the retropatellar space with constant negative pressure.
- Stop advancing once synovial fluid is aspirated; fill syringe with fluid; grasp needle with a hemostat to remove syringe; connect another syringe and continue aspirating until joint is dry.
- Remove needle and apply bandage.

TECHNIQUE FOR SHOULDER ARTHROCENTESIS

- Position: sitting position with arm at side and hand on lap (anterior approach) or with arm across waist (posterior approach).
- Sterile prep and drape of the shoulder.
- Anesthetize the skin and subcutaneous tissues at the insertion site.
- Anterior approach (**Figure 26-2**):
  - Insertion site is a thumb-width inferior and 1 cm lateral to the coracoid process.
  - Advance 20-gauge needle slightly superolaterally toward medial humeral head.

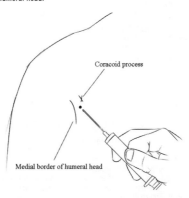

FIGURE 26-2. Glenohumeral Joint Arthrocentesis-Anterior Approach
Adapted from Tallia AF, Cardone DA. Diagnostic and Therapeutic Injection of the Shoulder Region. *Amer Fam Physician.* 2003; 67(6): 1273, Figure 1A.

The insertion site is 1 cm inferior and 1 cm lateral to the coracoid process. Direct needle superolaterally towards the medial humeral head.

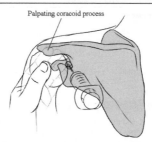

Palpating coracoid process

FIGURE 26-3. Glenohumeral Joint Arthrocentesis-Posterior Approach
Adapted from Zuber TJ. Knee Joint Aspiration and Injection. *Amer Fam Physician.* 2002;
66(8): 1273, Figure 1B.

Place the index finger of the non-syringe hand on the coracoid process. Insertion
site is 2 cm inferior and 1 cm medial to the posterolateral corner of acromion.
Aim the needle toward the coracoid process.

- Posterior approach (**Figure 26-3**):
  - Identify the posterolateral aspect of the acromion process.
  - Insertion site is 2 cm inferior and 1 cm medial to the posterolateral
    corner of acromion (depression felt).
  - Aim needle horizontally toward the coracoid process about 2–3 cm.
- Stop advancing once synovial fluid is aspirated; fill syringe with fluid;
  grasp needle with a hemostat to remove syringe; connect another
  syringe and continue aspirating until joint is dry.
- Remove needle and apply bandage.

TECHNIQUE FOR ELBOW ARTHROCENTESIS

- Position: flex elbow to 45°, pronate forearm; and place palm flat on a
  table.
- Sterile prep and drape of the elbow.
- Anesthetize the skin and subcutaneous tissues at the insertion site.
- A soft spot can be felt just proximal and posterior to the radial head.
  This is the insertion site where a 20-gauge needle is advanced medially
  into joint (**Figure 26-4**).
  - The center of a triangle formed by the lateral epicondyle, the radial
    head, and the olecranon is the insertion site (**Figure 26-5**).
- Stop advancing once synovial fluid is aspirated; fill syringe with fluid;
  grasp needle with a hemostat to remove syringe; connect another
  syringe and continue aspirating until joint is dry.

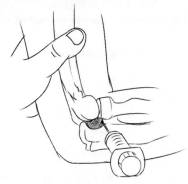

FIGURE 26-4. Elbow Arthrocentesis

Insert the needle just proximal and inferior to the radial head with the elbow held at 90°. Advance needle horizontally.

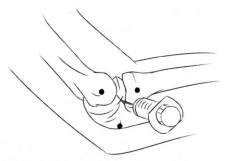

FIGURE 26-5. Elbow Arthrocentesis Landmarks
Adapted from Cardone DA, Tallia AF. Diagnostic and Therapeutic Injection of the Elbow Region. *Amer Fam Physician.* 2002; 66(11): 2098, Figure 1.

Insertion site is the center of a triangle formed by the lateral epicondyle, the radial head, and the olecranon.

SYNOVIAL FLUID ANALYSIS

- Cell count with differential, aerobic and anaerobic cultures, gram stain, and crystal analysis

COMPLICATIONS

- Joint or skin infection
- Intra-articular bleeding
- Allergic reaction to injected medication
- Vasovagal syncope
- Cartilage damage

CODING

20605	Arthrocentesis and/or injection of medium-sized joint (e.g., elbow)
20610	Arthrocentesis and/or injection of large joint (e.g., shoulder or knee)

REFERENCES

NEJM. 2006; 354: e19.
Amer Fam Physician. 2002; 66: 283.
Amer Fam Physician. 2002; 66: 1497–1500.
Amer Fam Physician. 2003; 67: 1271–1278.
Amer Fam Physician. 2003; 67: 2147–2152.
Amer Fam Physician. 2002; 66: 2097–2101.
Postgrad Med. 2001; 109: 123 and 157.

27 ■ JOINT INJECTIONS

INDICATIONS

- Joint pain
- Limited range of motion secondary to pain

CONTRAINDICATIONS

- Infection at injection site
- Hypersensitivity to anesthetic medication
- Joint instability due to ligamentous or tendinous injury
- Associated fracture or recent trauma to injection site
- Prosthetic joints
- Relative contraindications: diabetes or immunocompromised state; or coagulopathy

EQUIPMENT

- Povidone-iodine or chlorhexidine swabs
- Nonsterile and sterile gloves
- Single-dose medication vials
  - 1% lidocaine
  - Corticosteroid preparation
- 18-gauge, 27-gauge, and 22-gauge needles, 1 1/2 inches
- 3-ml syringe for anesthesia
- 10-ml syringe for injection
- 20–60-ml syringe for aspirating fluid
- Ethyl chloride spray
- Hemostat
- Sterile bandage

GENERAL TECHNIQUE FOR ALL INJECTIONS

- Organize all equipment and medications on a towel overlying Mayo stand.
- Place patient in optimum position.
- Mark insertion site with a needle guard, leaving an indented mark.
- Sterile prep of skin area.
- Anesthetize skin and underlying soft tissue with 1% lidocaine and a 27-gauge needle or Ethyl chloride spray.

- Direct 22-gauge needle toward target area; aspirate if target is a joint; or perform injection if target is a bursa or a tendon.
- If target is a joint:
  - Stop advancing once synovial fluid is aspirated; fill syringe with fluid; grasp needle with a hemostat to remove syringe; connect another syringe and continue aspirating until joint is dry; then remove syringe.
  - Attach new syringe prefilled with corticosteroid-anesthetic mixture to needle.
  - Perform injection.
- Place sterile bandage over injection site.

TECHNIQUE OF GLENOHUMERAL JOINT INJECTION

- Follow approach of glenohumeral joint arthrocentesis (anterior or posterior approach) as detailed on page 155, **Figure 26-2**, or page 156, **Figure 26-3**.
- Once joint fluid is aspirated dry, change syringe.
- Inject 6–9-ml medication mixture (**Table 27-1**).
- Avoid overhead activities for several days.

TECHNIQUE OF KNEE INJECTION

- Follow approach of knee joint aspiration (medial or lateral approach) as detailed on page 154, **Figure 26-1**.
- Once joint fluid is aspirated dry, change syringe.
- Inject 7–9-ml medication mixture (see **Table 27-1**).
- Avoid running for several days.

TECHNIQUE OF SUBACROMIAL BURSA INJECTION

- Identify lateral aspect of acromion.
- Mark spot 2–3 cm below middle of acromion (**Figure 27-1**).
- Direct needle slightly cephalad over the humeral head; advance 3 cm (**Figure 27-2**).
- Inject 6–9 ml medication mixture (see **Table 27-1**).
  - If resistance is felt during injection, withdraw needle 2 mm and continue injection.
  - Fan out injection.
- Avoid overhead activities for several days.

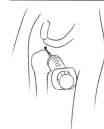

FIGURE 27-1. Insertion Site for Subacromial Bursa Injection

Adapted from Tallia AF, Cardone DA. Diagnostic and Therapeutic Injection of the Shoulder Region. *Amer Fam Physician.* 2003; 67(6): 1276, Figure 3.

The insertion site is 2–3 cm below the lateral aspect of the acromion.

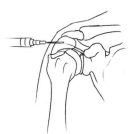

FIGURE 27-2. Lateral Approach to Subacromial Bursa Injection

Adapted from Weiss LD, Silver JK, Lennard TA, et al. *Easy Injections.* Philadelphia, PA: Butterworth-Heinemann; 2007: 86, Figure 5-1.

Direct needle slightly cephalad over the humeral head and advance ~3 cm.

TABLE 27-1. Corticosteroids for Joint Injections

Site	1% lidocaine	Corticosteroid*
Glenohumeral joint	5–7 ml	Methylprednisolone 40–60 mg (1–1.5 ml) Betamethasone 6–12 mg (1–2 ml)
Subacromial space	5–7 ml	Methylprednisolone 40–60 mg (1–1.5 ml) Betamethasone 6–12 mg (1–2 ml)
Knee joint	5–7 ml	Methylprednisolone 40–60 mg (1–1.5 ml) Betamethasone 12 mg (2 ml)
Greater trochanteric bursa	3–5 ml	Methylprednisolone 40 mg (1 ml) Betamethasone 6 mg (1 ml)6
Lateral epicondyle	3–5 ml	Methylprednisolone 20 mg (0.5 ml) Betamethasone 3 mg (0.5 ml)

*Equivalent amounts of triamcinolone or dexamethasone may be used.
Source: Data from *Amer Fam Physician.* 2003; 67: 1271–1278, *Amer Fam Physician.* 2003; 67: 2147–2152, and *Amer Fam Physician.* 1991; 44: 1690.

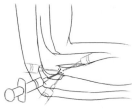

FIGURE 27-3. Lateral Epicondyle Injection
Adapted from Cardone DA, Tallia AF. Diagnostic and Therapeutic Injection of the Elbow Region. *Amer Fam Physician.* 2002; 66(11): 2099, Figure 3.

Inject just distal to the lateral epicondyle at the point of maximal tenderness; fan out the injection; avoid injecting directly into the tendon.

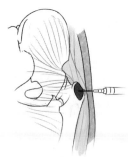

FIGURE 27-4. Trochanteric Bursa Injection
Adapted from Cardone DA, Tallia AF. Diagnostic and Therapeutic Injections of the Hip and Knee. *Amer Fam Physician.* 2003; 67(10): 2149, Figure 1.

Insert needle perpendicular to skin at the point of maximal tenderness until bone is reached; withdraw needle 2 mm and then inject solution.

TECHNIQUE FOR LATERAL EPICONDYLE INJECTION

- Flex elbow to 90° and pronate forearm with arm resting on a pillow over the body.
- Identify the radial head just distal to lateral epicondyle.
- Insertion site is the point of maximal tenderness, usually just distal to epicondyle (**Figure 27-3**).
- Use 22-gauge needle and inject 3.5–5.5 ml medication mixture in fan-like distribution just above tendon insertion (see **Table 27-1**).
  - Avoid direct tendon injection; if resistance is felt, withdraw needle 1 mm.
- Avoid heavy lifting for several days.

TECHNIQUE FOR TROCHANTERIC BURSA INJECTION

- Place patient in lateral decubitus position with affected side up.
- The point of maximal tenderness is at the greater trochanter, the bony protruberance along the lateral side of the proximal femur.
- Insert a 22-gauge needle perpendicular to skin at point of maximal tenderness until bone is reached; withdraw needle 2 mm (**Figure 27-4**).
- Inject 4–6 ml medication mixture (see **Table 27-1**).
- Avoid repetitive bending or running for several days.

POST-PROCEDURE CARE

- Ice area for 15 minutes several times a day for first 24–48 hours.
- After 24–48 hours, begin local heat and gentle stretching/range-of-motion exercises.

COMPLICATIONS

- Vasovagal syncope
- Anaphylaxis
- Post-injection flare (2–10% incidence)
- Subcutaneous or fat atrophy
- Skin hypopigmentation
- Steroid "chalk" calcification
- Steroid arthropathy
- Infection

CODING

20610	Injection of major joint (e.g., glenohumeral or knee) or bursa (e.g., subacromial or trochanteric bursae)
20550	Injection of tendon sheath (e.g., lateral epicondyle)

REFERENCES

J Clin Rheum. 2004; 10: 123–124.
Amer Fam Physician. 2003; 67: 1271–1278.
Amer Fam Physician. 2003; 67: 2147–2152.
Amer Fam Physician. 2002; 66: 283–289.
Int J Clin Pract. 2005; 59: 1178–1186.
Amer Fam Physician. 2002; 66: 2097–2101.
Clev Clin J Med. 2007; 74: 473–488.

SECTION XII

PULMONARY PROCEDURES

INDICATIONS

- Evaluation of unexplained dyspnea
- Evaluation of chronic cough
- Evaluation of unexplained hypoxia
- Evaluation of unexplained hypercapnia
- Evaluation of unexplained polycythemia
- Evaluation of abnormal chest x-ray
- To assess pulmonary reserve in patients with neuromuscular disorders
- Preoperative pulmonary evaluation
- To follow patients with chronic lung disease
- **Not** indicated for screening *asymptomatic* adults at risk for COPD

CONTRAINDICATIONS

- Patient is uncooperative or unable to follow directions
- Moderate–severe respiratory distress
- Severe nausea/vomiting
- Acute vertigo
- Hemoptysis of unclear etiology
- Pneumothorax
- Abdominal, thoracic, or ocular surgery within 8 weeks
- Recent MI or unstable angina within 8 weeks

EQUIPMENT

- Comfortable chair
- Spirometer
- Nose clips
- Disposable mouthpieces

TECHNIQUE

- Calibrate spirometer.
- Apply nose clip.
- Have patient take a few normal spontaneous breaths in and out through the mouth.

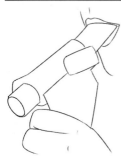

FIGURE 28-1. Use of a Spirometer

The patient takes a deep breath in, then seals mouth around the mouthpiece and blows out as fast and long as possible.

- Then have patient take in as deep a breath as possible, then seal mouth around mouthpiece and blow out as fast and long as possible (**Figure 28-1**).
  - Encourage patient to continue breathing until FVC curve flattens out (usually 5–6 seconds).
- Then patient breathes in as deeply as possible.
- Repeat this sequence three times.
- Perform testing pre-bronchodilator and post-bronchodilator (to assess for reversibility).

ACCEPTABILITY CRITERIA

- Spirograms must be free from coughing
- No early termination of breath
- No variability of effort
- No air leak
- Satisfactory exhalation: six seconds or plateau in volume-time curve
- Reproducibility criteria are met

REPRODUCIBILITY CRITERIA

- Two largest FVC within 0.15 L of each other
- Two largest FEV_1 within 0.15 L of each other

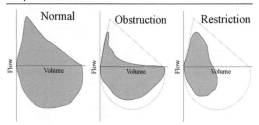

FIGURE 28-2. Spirograms and Flow Volume Curves
Adapted from Gold WM. Pulmonary Function Testing. In: Murray JF, Nadel JA, Mason RJ, et al., eds. *Textbook of Respiratory Medicine.* 3rd ed. Philadelphia, PA: Saunders; 2000: 805, Figure 28.21.

(A) Normal spirogram; (B) Obstructive ventilatory defect; (C) Restrictive ventilatory defect.

INTERPRETATION OF RESULTS

- Flow volume curves (**Figure 28-2**)
- Interpretation of TLC, and FVC in restrictive lung disease (**Table 28-1**)
- Interpretation of FEV_1 in obstructive lung disease (**Table 28-2**)
- FEV_1/FVC ratio will be normal in restrictive lung disease
- FEV_1/FVC ratio will be < 70% in obstructive lung disease

TABLE 28-1. Grading of Spirometric Abnormalities in Restrictive Lung Disease

Severity of Restriction	% Predicted TLC	% Predicted FVC
Mild	70–80%	70–80%
Moderate	60–69%	60–69%
Moderate–severe	50–59%	50–59%
Severe	35–49%	35–49%
Very severe	< 35%	< 35%

TLC = total lung capacity, FVC = forced vital capacity
Source: Modified from Grading of PFT Abnormalities. In: Esherick JS. *Tarascon Primary Care Pocketbook.* 3rd ed. Sudbury, MA: Jones & Bartlett Learning; 2010: 148.

TABLE 28-2. Grading of Spirometric Abnormalities in Obstructive Lung Disease

Severity of Obstruction	% Predicted FEV$_1$
Mild	70–80%
Moderate	60–69%
Moderate–severe	50–59%
Severe	35–49%
Very severe	< 35%

TLC = total lung capacity, FVC = forced vital capacity, LLN = lower limit of normal
Source: Modified from Grading of PFT Abnormalities. In: Esherick JS. *Tarascon Primary Care Pocketbook.* 3rd ed. Sudbury, MA: Jones & Bartlett Learning; 2010: 148.

COMPLICATIONS

- None

CODING

94010	Spirometry, including graphic record, total and timed vital capacity, expiratory flow rate measurements, with or without maximal voluntary ventilation
94060	Spirometry before and after bronchodilator therapy
94375	Flow-volume loop interpretation

REFERENCES

Amer Fam Physician. 2004; 69: 1107–1114.
Chest. 2005; 128: 2443–2447.
Ann Intern Med. 2008; 148: 529–534.
Esherick, JS. Tarascon *Primary Care Pocketbook*, 3rd Ed. Sudbury, MA: Jones & Bartlett Learning: 2010: 148.
Gold WM. Pulmonary Function Testing. In: Murray, JF, Nadal JA, Mason RJ et al., eds. *Textbook of Respiratory Medicine*, 3rd ed. Philadelphia, PA: Saunders: 2000: 805.

29 ■ THORACENTESIS

- **Diagnostic Thoracentesis**
  - Work-up of unexplained pleural effusion
  - Rule out empyema or infected parapneumonic effusion
- **Therapeutic Thoracentesis**
  - To relieve dyspnea and improve oxygenation

CONTRAINDICATIONS

- **Absolute Contraindications**
  - Uncooperative patient
  - Overlying skin infection
  - Ruptured diaphragm
- **Relative Contraindications**
  - Small pleural effusion (≤ 1 cm on lateral decubitus chest x-ray)
  - Mechanical ventilation
  - Coagulopathy (INR > 1.8 or PTT >1.5–2 x upper limit of normal)
  - Thrombocytopenia (Platelets < 50K)
  - Severe uremia

EQUIPMENT

- Numerous prepackaged thoracentesis trays are available
- Surgeon's cap
- Face mask with eye protection
- Sterile gloves and gown
- Sterile prep: chlorhexidine or povidone-iodine swabs
- 10-ml labeled syringe with needles for anesthesia
- 1% lidocaine with or without epinephrine
- 2-inch 22-gauge finder needle
- 3-inch 16-gauge angiocatheter or a thoracentesis-specific catheter (e.g., Pleura-Seal Thoracentesis kit or Saf-T-Centesis Catheter Drainage tray)
- 60-ml syringe for aspiration of pleural fluid
- Three-way stopcock
- High-pressure drainage tubing
- Sterile labeled specimen tubes

- One or two large evacuated containers
- May need a lithium heparin tube on ice (pleural fluid pH sampling)
- May need aerobic and anaerobic culture bottles (if infection possible)
- Sterile bandage

TECHNIQUE

- Informed consent.
- Have patient seated at the edge of the bed with arms draped over a table.
- Percuss/auscultate out superior margin of effusion (or identify with ultrasound).
  - For large pleural effusions, typically use the 8th intercostal space in the mid-scapular line (**Figure 29-1**).
    - 8th intercostal space lies immediately below the scapular tip.
  - If the extent of the pleural effusion is equivocal, consider using ultrasound to mark the insertion site.
  - Assure that the ultrasound is performed in the same position as the planned procedure.
- Perform a "time out" and mark site after rechecking a chest x-ray to confirm correct side.

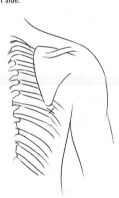

FIGURE 29-1. Thoracentesis Landmarks

The scapular tip is the primary landmark for a thoracentesis using a posterior approach in the sitting position. The insertion site is usually above the ninth rib in the mid-scapular line.

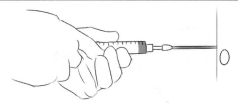

FIGURE 29-2. Advancing Thoracentesis Needle Into Pleural Space

A thoracentesis needle is inserted over the rib with constant negative pressure until fluid is aspirated.

- Anesthetize skin, periosteum, and pleura **over the rib**.
- Advance 1.5-inch 22-gauge finder needle with constant aspiration until fluid return.
  - Memorize depth required to enter pleural space.
- Advance thoracentesis needle until fluid is aspirated (**Figure 29-2**).
- Advance catheter through needle or over the needle (**Figure 29-3**) and aspirate 50 ml pleural fluid for diagnostic studies (**Figure 29-4**).
- Withdraw needle, leaving the catheter in place.
  - If catheter-through-needle system, apply a clamp at the needle and catheter juncture.

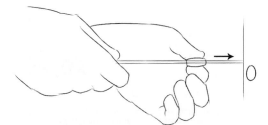

FIGURE 29-3. Advancing Thoracentesis Catheter Over Needle

Once fluid is obtained, the needle is held stationary as the catheter is advanced over the needle. The needle is then withdrawn.

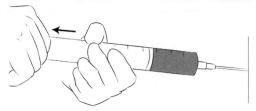

FIGURE 29-4. Aspiration of Pleural Fluid

A 60-ml syringe is attached to the thoracentesis catheter to withdraw pleural fluid for analysis.

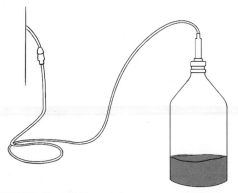

FIGURE 29-5. Therapeutic Thoracentesis

Suction tubing can be attached to the thoracentesis catheter and the other end inserted into an evacuated container for rapid aspiration of fluid.

- Attach tubing to suction canister for therapeutic thoracentesis (**Figure 29-5**).
  - Stop aspiration for aspiration of air, worsening dyspnea, severe chest pain, or persistent coughing.
  - Alternatively, a three-way stopcock may be used to aspirate fluid by hand into a 60-ml syringe and then emptied into an in-line collection bag.
- Check a chest x-ray to check for a pneumothorax.

PLEURAL FLUID ANALYSIS (TABLE 29-1)

- Common causes of transudates: CHF, nephrotic syndrome, hepatic hydrothorax, +/- PE
- Causes of exudates: empyema, cancer, viral pneumonitis, pleural Tb, S/P CABG, SLE, PE
- **Routine Studies**: cell count with differential; protein; albumin; LDH; glucose; gram stain; and bedside inoculation of aerobic and anaerobic culture bottles
  - Confirm that serum protein and LDH have been drawn simultaneously for comparison.
- **Optional Studies if Clinically Indicated**: pleural fluid pH (lithium heparin tube on ice); cytology; CEA (Ratio of pleural fluid CEA/serum CEA ≥ 20 = lung CA); triglycerides: > 110 mg/dl = chylothorax; AFB RNA by PCR, AFB culture +/- adenosine deaminase level

COMPLICATIONS

- Pneumothorax (incidence about 6%)
  - Tube thoracostomy is indicated if the pneumothorax is symptomatic, is causing clinical instability or is greater than 15% in size
- Reexpansion pulmonary edema if > 1500 ml pleural fluid removed at one time (2.5% risk)
- Local infection (2% risk)
- Laceration of intercostal artery causing a hemothorax (1.2%)
- Shearing of the catheter
- Injury to spleen, liver, diaphragm, or lung
  - Avoid entry sites below 8th intercostal space in midscapular line unless the thoracentesis is ultrasound-guided

TABLE 29-1. Pleural Fluid Classification

Test	Transudate	Exudate
Pleural fluid protein/serum protein	< 0.5	≥ 0.5‡
Pleural fluid LDH (IU)	< 200	>2/3 upper limit normal‡
Pleural fluid LDH/serum LDH	< 0.6	≥ 0.6‡
Serum-effusion albumin gradient	> 1.2 gm/dl¥	≤ 1.2 gm/dl
Pleural fluid glucose (mg/dl)	> 60	≤ 60*

‡—Light's criteria: only one test needs to be abnormal to classify as an exudate
*: glucose < 60 suggests cancer, tuberculosis, empyema, SLE, rheumatoid lung
¥: Useful to identify transudates misclassified as exudates
  • Pleural fluid lymphocytosis > 50%: 90–96% from either malignancy or tuberculosis
  • Pleural fluid pH < 7.2: empyema, malignancy, rheumatoid or lupus effusion, pleural tuberculosis, ruptured esophagus or urinothorax
  • Bloody fluid: trauma, malignancy, pulmonary embolus, or tuberculosis
Source: Data from Porcel JM, Light RW. Diagnostic Approach to Pleural Effusions in Adults. *Amer Fam Physician.* 2006; 73: 1211–1220.

CODING

32421   Thoracentesis, puncture of pleural cavity for aspiration, initial or subsequent

76942   Ultrasound guidance for thoracentesis

REFERENCES

NEJM. 2001; 345: 756–759.
NEJM. 2002; 346: 1971–1977.
NEJM. 2006; 355: e16–e19.
Amer Fam Physician. 2006; 73: 1211–1220.

30 ■ BASICS OF MECHANICAL VENTILATION

- **Choose the mode of ventilation**
  - Assist control (AC) if very limited patient effort or heavy sedation
  - Synchronized intermittent mandatory ventilation (SIMV) if some respiratory effort or patient-ventilator dyssynchrony on AC
  - Pressure control (PC) if patient is pressure limiting on the ventilator
- **Settings for oxygenation**
  - Initial FiO_2 0.8–1.0; adjust according to oxygen saturation (SaO_2)
  - Initial positive end-expiratory pressure (PEEP) 5 cm H_2O; adjust according to FiO_2 (see PEEP-FiO_2 algorithm below)
  - Aim for $SaO_2 \geq 90\%$, $PaO_2 \geq 60$ mm Hg
  - Aim to titrate $FiO_2 \leq 0.6$
- **Settings for ventilation**
  - Tidal volume: 6–8 ml/kg predicted body weight (PBW)
    - PBW for men (kg) = $50 + [2.3 \times$ (height in inches minus 60)]
    - PBW for women (kg) = $45.5 + [2.3 \times$ (height in inches minus 60)]
  - Ventilator rate: 10–14/minute; adjust based on $PaCO_2$ and pH
    - Consider initial rate of 20–24/minute in acute respiratory distress syndrome (ARDS)
    - Can increase rate to 35 breaths/minute if necessary
  - Keep plateau pressure ≤ 30 cm H_2O
- **Additional ventilator settings**
  - Triggering sensitivity: adjust to minimize patient effort
  - I:E ratio: initially 1:2; decrease inspiratory time for severe bronchospasm; and can increase inspiratory time for refractory hypoxia
  - Pressure support: if SIMV mode, can adjust between 6–20 cm H_2O titrated to patient comfort
  - Lung protective ventilation is indicated for ARDS/acute lung injury or severe sepsis/septic shock
  - Allow permissive hypercapnia as long as patient has no increased intracranial pressure
  - May use sodium bicarbonate drip if necessary to keep pH > 7.15
- **Monitoring During Mechanical Ventilation**
  - Continuous cardiopulmonary monitor
  - Ventilator: tidal volume, minute volume, airway pressures, serial arterial blood gases
  - End-tidal carbon dioxide (E_TCO_2) monitors desirable for ventilator weaning

GENERAL GUIDELINES FOR MECHANICAL VENTILATION

- Adjust ventilation by changing minute volume
  - Minute volume = tidal volume × respiratory rate
- Ventilate to pH, not to $PaCO_2$
- Improving oxygenation: increase FiO_2, PEEP or inspiratory time (if refractory hypoxia) (**Table 30-1**)
- Avoid paralytics if possible
- Continuous sedation titrated to patient comfort (control pain, anxiety, and delirium)
  - Analgesic options: opioids (e.g., fentanyl); dexmedetomidine; or ketamine
  - Anxiolysis options: benzodiazepines (e.g., lorazepam or midazolam); propofol; ketamine; or dexmedetomidine
  - Management of delirium: antipsychotics
  - Titrate analgesia and sedation based on a standard sedation scale (e.g., Ramsey Sedation scale, Sedation Agitation Scale, or Richmond Agitation-Sedation Scale [RASS])
  - Daily interruption of continuous sedation and assessment of readiness to extubate
- Use an active weaning protocol including daily spontaneous breathing trials (**Figure 30-1**)
- Prophylaxis: head of bed elevation to 45°, chlorhexidine oral rinses, low-molecular weight or unfractionated heparin, sequential compression devices, and proton pump inhibitor

COMPLICATIONS OF MECHANICAL VENTILATION

- Pneumothorax or pneumomediastinum (especially if plateau pressure exceeds 30 cm H_2O)
- Ventilator-associated lung injury (especially if Vt > 10 ml/kg PBW)
- Hypotension (especially if PEEP > 10 cm H_2O)
- Ventilator-associated pneumonia
- Stress gastric ulcers
- Venous thromboembolism
- Sinusitis
- Tracheal stenosis (if prolonged endotracheal intubation)
- Tracheomalacia (if prolonged endotracheal intubation)

TABLE 30-1. PEEP-FiO₂ Algorithm for Lung Protective Ventilation

FiO_2	.3	.4	.4	.5	.5	.6	.7	.7	.7	.8	.9	.9	.9	1.0	1.0	1.0	1.0
PEEP*	5	5	8	8	10	10	10	12	14	14	14	16	18	18	20	22	24

*: PEEP measured in cm H_2O

Source: Data from ARDS Clinical Trial Network. *N. Engl J. Med.* 2004; 351(4): 327–336 and *N Engl J Med.* 2000; 342(18): 1301–1308.

Patient is ready for a Spontaneous Breathing Trial if they meet the following criteria:

- Awake, cooperative and follows commands
- Good gag reflex
- Strong cough
- Minimal secretions
- Hemodynamically stable off vasopressors
- The underlying disease leading to intubation has improved
- Spontaneously breathing on PEEP<5-8
- PaO_2/FiO_2 ratio≥150-200 (or SaO_2≥90% with FiO_2≤0.4)
- Systemic pH≥7.25
- Minute ventilation<15 L/minute
- Rapid shallow breath index (f/Vt) <105 breaths/min/L

Spontaneous Breathing Trial (SBT)
- Settings: T-piece or CPAP with PEEP 5 cm H_2O & PS 6-8 cm H_2O
- Duration: 30-120 minutes
- Patient passes SBT if:
  - RR≤35
  - HR<120-140/minute
  - SBP>90 and <180 mmHg
  - SaO_2≥90% or PaO_2≥55 mmHg on FiO_2≤0.4
  - V_T≥4 mL/kg predicted body weight or ≥325 mL (in adults)
  - $PaCO_2$ increase<10 mmHg
  - Absence of agitation, diaphoresis or increased work of breathing

← Daily SBT trials →

Resume Mechanical Ventilation
- Search for causes of failure
  - Malnutrition
  - Electrolyte abnormalities
  - Cardiopulmonary disease
  - Mucous plugging
  - Oversedation
  - Neurologic dysfunction
  - Underlying disease necessitating mechanical ventilation has not sufficiently improved
- Resume a non-fatiguing mode of ventilation

Fails SBT →

Extubate if successful SBT

Daily ventilator weaning
- Pressure support weaning
  - PEEP 5-8 cm H_2O
  - PS 6-20 cm H_2O to keep respiratory rate<30/minute
  - Gradually wean PS by 2-4 cm H_2O as tolerated
- If patient is unable to tolerate PS ventilation, use SIMV mode
  - Slowly reduce backup rate as tolerated

FiO_2, fraction of inspired oxygen; HR, heart rate; $PaCO_2$, partial pressure arterial carbon dioxide; PaO_2, partial pressure arterial oxygen; PEEP, positive end-expiratory pressure; PS, pressure support; RR, respiratory rate; SaO_2, arterial oxygen saturation; SBP, systolic blood pressure; SIMV, synchronized intermittent mandatory ventilation; V_T, tidal volume.

FIGURE 30-1. Weaning and Liberation from Mechanical Ventilators
Adapted from Robertson TE, Mann HJ, Hyzy R, et al. Multicenter implementation of a consensus-developed, evidence-based, spontaneous breathing trial protocol. *Crit Care Med.* 2008; 36(10): 2754, Figure 1.

CODING

94002	Ventilator assist and management, hospital, initial day
94003	Ventilator assist and management, hospital, subsequent days
94005	Home ventilator management care plan oversight, ≥ 30 minutes

REFERENCES

NEJM. 2004; 351(4): 327–336.
NEJM. 2000; 342(18): 1301–1308.
Chest. 2001; 120: 375S–395S.
Crit Care Med. 2008; 36: 706–714.
NEJM. 2001; 344(26): 1986–1996.
Crit Care Med. 2006; 34: 2541–2546.
Crit Care Med. 2008; 36: 2753.
J Trauma. 2007; 63: 945–950.

31 ■ TUBE THORACOSTOMY

INDICATIONS

- Hemothorax
- Chylothorax
- Pneumothorax
  - Symptomatic or clinical instability or on mechanical ventilation
  - Recurrent pneumothorax
  - Small spontaneous secondary pneumothorax
  - Asymptomatic large primary pneumothorax
    - Chest wall-to-lung margin ≥ 1 cm or apex-to-cupola ≥ 2 cm
  - Associated with penetrating chest trauma
- Esophageal rupture with leak into pleural space
- Empyema or complicated parapneumonic effusions
- Use for chemical pleurodesis in malignant effusions
- Prevention of hydrothorax after cardiothoracic surgery, thoracotomy, or lung resection
- Drainage of recurrent or refractory pleural effusions

CONTRAINDICATIONS

- None if the procedure is emergent
- Contraindications to semi-elective chest tube placement
  - Coagulopathy
  - Thrombocytopenia (Platelets < 50,000)
  - Pleural effusion secondary to pleural tuberculosis
  - Overlying skin infection
  - Known pleural adhesions or history of a pleurodesis
  - Known or suspected mesothelioma
  - Caution if pleural effusion is loculated (consider ultrasound guidance)

EQUIPMENT

- Sterile gown and gloves
- Cap and mask
- Sterile towels
- 10-ml syringe with 25-gauge and 22-gauge needles
- 1% lidocaine +/– epinephrine

- 2 long curved Kelly clamps
- No. 10 blade on scalpel
- Sterile prep: chlorhexidine or povidone-iodine swabs
- 5-in-1 connector
- Chest tube
  - 10F–14F for primary spontaneous pneumothorax
  - 18F–22F for secondary spontaneous pneumothorax
  - 24F–28F for large air leaks or mechanical ventilation or tension pneumothorax
  - 32F–36F for empyema or infected parapneumonic effusion
  - 32F–36F for traumatic pneumothorax or hemothorax
- Needle driver
- 1-0 silk suture or equivalent (two packs)
- Petrolatum gauze
- Sterile pack of 4 × 4-inch gauze pads
- Suture scissors
- Foam tape
- Pleural drainage system with a waterseal compartment appropriately filled

TECHNIQUE

- Informed consent.
- Perform a "time out" and mark site after rechecking chest x-ray to confirm correct side.
- Consider procedural sedation in a monitored bed for a nonemergent tube thoracostomy.
- Positioning:
  - Semi-recumbent at 45°, if possible, with ipsilateral arm secured over head (**Figure 31-1**)
- Wash hands and then don sterile attire.
- Insertion site:
  - 4th–5th intercostal space in mid-axillary line
  - Lateral to the pectoralis major muscle and anterior to the latissimus dorsi
    - In ♂, nipple is at 4th intercostal space (ICS)
    - In ♀, 4th ICS is 3 fingers above xiphoid notch carried laterally to axillary line
- Anesthetize skin overlying 4th–5th ICS, underlying soft tissue, the 5th–6th rib periosteum, and the parietal pleura immediately over 5th–6th rib (**Figure 31-2**).
  - Max dose is 4.5 mg/kg lidocaine and 7 mg/kg lidocaine with epinephrine
  - 1% lidocaine = 10 mg/ml
- Measure approximate distance chest tube can be advanced.

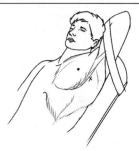

FIGURE 31-1. Proper Positioning for Chest Tube Placement

Adapted from Dev SP, Nascimiento B Jr, Simone C, et al. Chest-Tube Insertion. *N Engl J Med.* 2007; 357(15): e16, Figure 1.

The patient is placed in a semi-upright position with the ipsilateral arm secured over the head. The incision site is typically one interspace below the nipple in the mid-axillary line.

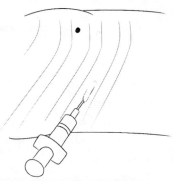

FIGURE 31-2. Local Anesthesia for Chest Tube Placement

1% lidocaine is used to anesthetize the skin, rib periosteum and the pleura for chest tube placement.

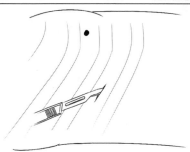

FIGURE 31-3. Skin Incision for Chest Tube Placement

A 3–4 cm skin incision is made parallel to the ribs in the 4th or 5th intercostal space.

- 3 cm incision parallel to ribs in 4th–5th ICS (**Figure 31-3**).
- Bluntly dissect with Kelly clamp over 5th–6th rib and enter pleural space (**Figure 31-4**).
- Spread clamp tips wide and withdraw clamp.
- Use finger to probe opening, feel the lung and **assure no adhesions.**
- Grasp chest tube with Kelly clamp and guide tube next to finger and into pleural space as finger retracted (**Figure 31-5**).
- Open Kelly clamp and advance chest tube.
- In most adults, chest tubes can be advanced 8–12 cm beyond the tube's last hole.
- Simple interrupted "stay" sutures on each side of tube (**Figure 31-6**).
- Wrap excess suture around tube to secure in place.
- Cover insertion site with petrolatum gauze; then place sterile 4 × 4s over insertion site and tape in place.
- Connect chest tube to a pleural drainage system placed to −20 cm wall suction.
- Chest radiograph to confirm correct positioning of chest tube.
- Single dose of cefazolin 1 gm IV indicated if chest tube is placed for trauma or in emergent settings.

CHEST TUBE TROUBLESHOOTING

- Persistent Pneumothorax
  - Assure that all connections are tight and secure.
  - No kinks in tubing and wall suction is on and functional.

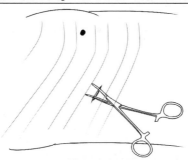

FIGURE 31-4. Blunt Dissection During Chest Tube Placement

A curved Kelly clamp is used to bluntly dissect over the rib superior to the skin incision and through the pleura into the pleural space.

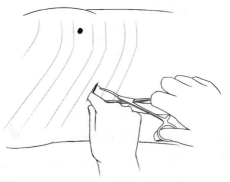

FIGURE 31-5. Chest Tube Insertion

A chest tube is inserted alongside a finger that is positioned in the pleural space. Initially, the chest tube is advanced with the aid of a curved Kelly clamp. Once the clamp is near the pleural opening, the finger is withdrawn and the chest tube is advanced into the pleural space.

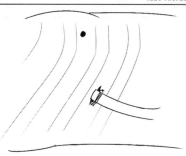

FIGURE 31-6. Securing Chest Tube with Suture

Chest tube secured with stay sutures on each side of the chest tube.

- Check for air leak.
- Consider increasing the flow of oxygen to help expedite lung reinflation.
- Increase suction to −25 cm H$_2$O if no air leak.
- Cardiac dysrhythmias and left chest tube
  - Pull back chest tube 2–3 cm.
- Causes of a persistent air leak
  - Leak in system (stops if tube clamped between leak and water seal)
  - Air entering around chest tube
  - Chest tube migration with the proximal side port outside the chest wall
  - Bronchopleural fistula
  - Tracheal or bronchial disruption (usually very large air leak)

DISCONTINUATION OF CHEST TUBES

- Pneumothorax
  - Can place chest tube to water seal once lung is reinflated **and no air leak**
  - Discontinue chest tube if lung completely inflated on water seal for 6–12 hours
  - Check a chest x-ray 12–24 hours after discontinuation (3 hours if on a ventilator)
- Hemothorax or non-infected pleural effusions
  - Can discontinue once drainage is less than 100–200 ml/day

- Empyema or infected parapneumonic effusion
  - Can discontinue once drainage is serous and output is less than 50–100 mL/day
- Technique
  - Positioning: semi-upright at 45°.
  - Cut sutures attached to the chest tube.
  - Briskly remove the chest tube at end-inspiration.
  - Cover the site with petrolatum gauze and then sterile 4 × 4 gauze.
  - Tape dressing in place with foam tape.
  - Repeat chest x-ray in 12–24 hours (three hours if patient on ventilator).
  - Remove dressing in 48 hours.
  - Discontinue skin sutures in 10 days.

COMPLICATIONS OF TUBE THORACOSTOMY

- **Major Complications**
  - Injury to liver, spleen, diaphragm, intestines, aorta, heart, lung, or intercostal arteries
  - Lung parenchyma perforation
  - Empyema
  - Cardiac dysrhythmias (from abutting left chest tube)
  - Open or tension pneumothorax
  - Laceration of long thoracic nerve
- **Minor Complications**
  - Subcutaneous emphysema
  - Subcutaneous placement of tube
  - Persistent air leak
  - Localized infection at insertion site
  - Dislodged chest tube
  - Reexpansion pulmonary edema (2.5% incidence)
    - Occurs with rapid removal of > 1.5 liters of fluid (or less in children)

CODING

32551   Tube thoracostomy, with or without water seal

REFERENCES

NEJM. 2000; 342: 868.
NEJM. 2007; 357: e15.
Thorax, 2003; 58 (Supp 2): S1.
J Amer Coll Surg. 2002; 195: 658.
Chest. 2001; 119: 590–602.
J Trauma. 2000; 48: 753–759.

SECTION XIII

VASCULAR PROCEDURES

32 ■ CENTRAL VENOUS ACCESS

INDICATIONS FOR CENTRAL VENOUS CATHETERS

- Central venous pressure (CVP) monitoring
- Central parenteral nutrition infusion
- No peripheral access
- Temporary hemodialysis access
- Plasmapheresis
- Infusion of vasopressor medications
- Infusion of potentially caustic solutions: various chemotherapy meds or hypertonic saline
- Introducer access for a pulmonary artery catheter or transvenous pacemaker
- Emergency venous access during a cardiac arrest

CONTRAINDICATIONS OF CENTRAL VENOUS CATHETER PLACEMENT

- Patient refuses or is too combative
- Venous thrombosis of target vein
- Superior vena cava syndrome (for subclavian or internal jugular vein catheterization)
- Inferior vena cava filter (relative contraindication for femoral vein catheterization)
- Soft tissue infection, burns or abrasions involving the entry site for central line
- Trauma to the site
- Uncorrected bleeding diathesis AND noncompressible vessel (subclavian vessels)
  - PTT > 1.5 × upper limit of normal
  - INR > 1.5 in patient on warfarin
  - Platelets < 50K
  - Uremia
  - Caution with chronic antiplatelet therapy

EQUIPMENT

- Sterile gown and gloves
- Mask with face shield
- Surgeon's cap
- Sterile prep: chlorhexidine or povidone-iodine swabs
- Sterile drape
- 5-ml syringe × 2

- 25-gauge and 22-gauge needles
- Sterile syringes filled with sterile saline
- 1% lidocaine for local anesthesia
- J-tipped flexible guidewire
- No. 11 scalpel
- Dilator
- Central venous catheter
- Silk or nylon suture
- Sterile occlusive dressing

GENERAL TECHNIQUE FOR CENTRAL LINE PLACEMENT IN ALL LOCATIONS

- Informed consent.
- Perform a "time out" to confirm the correct patient, side, and procedure.
- Wash hands and then don a surgeon's cap and mask, and a sterile gown and gloves.
- Wide sterile prep of the procedure area with either chlorhexidine or povidone-iodine.
  - Chlorhexidine is preferred to povidone-iodine.
- Wide sterile drape of the procedure area.
- Flush all catheter ports with sterile saline.
- 15–20° Trendelenberg position for internal jugular or subclavian vein catheterizations.
- Modified Seldinger technique utilized for placement of central venous catheter:
  - Anesthetize skin and underlying soft tissue.
  - Advance introducer needle connected to syringe under constant negative pressure until a flash of blood is seen (**Figure 32-1**).
  - Disconnect syringe from needle and assure non-pulsatile, purple venous blood return.
  - Introduce guidewire through the needle with J tip directed toward the heart to a depth of 20 cm (**Figure 32-2**).
  - Withdraw needle, leaving wire in place.
  - Use scalpel to nick the skin over the wire (**Figure 32-3**).
  - Place dilator over the wire and advance dilator through the skin and into the vein with a rotating motion (**Figure 32-4**).
  - Withdraw the dilator, leaving the wire in place.
  - Introduce the central venous catheter over the wire (**Figure 32-5**).
  - Withdraw the wire into the catheter and grasp the wire tip beyond the most distal catheter port.
  - Advance the catheter over wire to the appropriate depth of insertion:
    - Right subclavian vein: 13–16 cm
    - Left subclavian vein: 14–17 cm
    - Right internal jugular vein: 12–14 cm
    - Left internal jugular vein: 13–16 cm

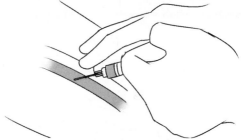

FIGURE 32-1. Cannulating Left Formal Vein

The fingers are palpating the artery and the introducer needle is advanced at a 45° angle to the skin until a flash of purple blood is obtained.

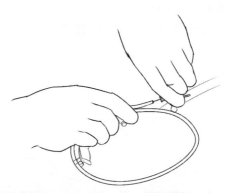

FIGURE 32-2. Threading the Wire Through the Introducer Needle

Once the vein is cannulated, the syringe is disconnected from the introducer needle to confirm the return of purple, nonpulsatile blood and then a flexible wire is advanced through the needle with the J tip directed toward the heart.

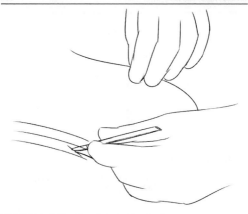

FIGURE 32-3. Nicking Skin with Scalpel Over the Wire

A scalpel is used to nick the skin over the wire after the needle is withdrawn from the wire. Always maintain control of guidewire.

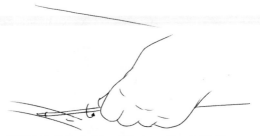

FIGURE 32-4. Dilating the Skin and Subcutaneous Tissue Over the Wire

A dilator is advanced over the wire with a twisting motion to dilate a tract through the skin, soft tissue, and vein. The dilator is then withdrawn over the wire, leaving the wire in place.

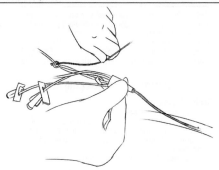

FIGURE 32-5. A Central Venous Catheter Is Introduced Over Wire

A triple-lumen catheter is inserted over wire and advanced to a predesignated depth of insertion. The wire is then withdrawn through the distal port of the catheter. Each catheter port will then be flushed with sterile saline.

- Withdraw the wire and cap the distal port.
- Flush all catheter ports again with sterile saline.
- Secure catheter in place with suture (**Figure 32-6**).
- Apply a clear, sterile dressing over catheter insertion site.

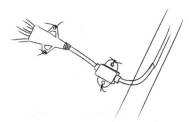

FIGURE 32-6. Securing the Central Venous Catheter In Place

A central venous catheter is secured in place in four locations with suture. A sterile, transparent occlusive dressing is then placed over the catheter at the insertion site.

- Check a chest x-ray after placement of a subclavian or internal jugular vein catheter to confirm appropriate catheter tip location and to check for a pneumothorax.
- Ultrasound guidance of internal jugular or femoral vein catheterization by experienced operators reduces the incidence of mechanical complications (relative risk 0.32), insertion attempts, and procedure time.

INTERNAL JUGULAR VEIN CATHETERS

- **Central Approach**
  - Landmarks (**Figure 32-7**)
    - Sternal and clavicular heads of sternocleidomastoid muscle form a triangle with the clavicle as the base of the triangle
    - Ipsilateral nipple (or midclavicular line in women)
  - Positioning
    - Turn head 30° to contralateral side

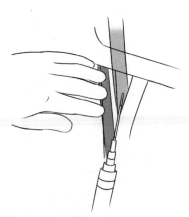

FIGURE 32-7. Central Approach to Internal Jugular Vein Catheterization

The fingers are overlying the carotid pulse. The anterior cervical triangle is bordered by the sternal and clavicular heads of the sternocleidomastoid muscle and inferiorly by the clavicle. The insertion site is 1 cm inferior to the apex of the triangle and just lateral to the carotid pulse. The needle is inserted at a 30–40° angle to the skin and aiming toward the ipsilateral nipple.

- Entry site and needle direction
  - Insert just below the apex of the triangle, 1 cm lateral to the carotid pulse.
  - Aim needle toward the ipsilateral nipple 30–45° to the skin.
  - Vein should be entered within 3 cm.
- **Posterior Approach**
  - Landmarks
    - Posterolateral border of the clavicular head of the sternocleido-mastoid muscle
    - Sternal notch
  - Positioning
    - Turn head 30° to contralateral side.
  - Entry site and needle direction
    - Entry site is just above where the external jugular vein crosses the posterolateral edge of the sternocleidomastoid muscle (about 5 cm above the clavicle).
    - Aim towards the sternal notch 15° anterior to horizontal.
    - Vein should be entered within 5 cm.

SUBCLAVIAN VEIN CATHETERS

- **Infraclavicular Approach**
  - Landmarks **(Figure 32-8)**
    - Curve of the clavicle (or intersection of clavicle and first rib)
    - Sternal notch
  - Positioning
    - Turn head 30° to contralateral side.
  - Entry site and needle direction
    - Entry site is 1 cm lateral and 0.5 cm inferior to the curve of clavicle.
    - Aim 1 finger-width above the sternal notch with needle as parallel to the bed as possible; may use thumb of non-syringe hand to help push needle under clavicle.
    - Vein should be entered within 5 cm.
- **Supraclavicular Approach**
  - Landmarks
    - Lateral boarder of the sternocleidomastoid muscle
    - Sternal notch and ipsilateral sternoclavicular joint
  - Positioning
    - Turn head 30° to contralateral side.
  - Entry site and needle direction
    - Entry site is 1 cm lateral and 1 cm cephalad from the point at which the clavicular head of the sternocleidomastoid muscle inserts onto the clavicle.
    - Aim needle toward sternal notch at an angle 10–15° anterior to the horizontal plane.
    - Vein should be entered within 2–3 cm.

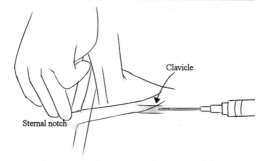

FIGURE 32-8. Infraclavicular Approach to Subclavian Vein Catheterization

Insertion site for infraclavicular subclavian line placement is 1 cm lateral and 0.5 cm inferior to the curve of the clavicle. The introducer needle is kept as parallel to the ground as possible and is directed toward the **tip** of the finger **that** is located in the sternal notch.

FEMORAL VEIN CATHETERS

- Landmarks (**Figure 32-9**)
  - Medial to femoral artery pulsation about 2 cm below inguinal ligament
  - Vein located 2/3 distance from anterior superior iliac spine to the pubic tubercle
- Positioning
  - Supine position with leg slightly abducted and toes pointing toward ceiling
- Entry site and needle direction
  - Entry site is 1 cm medial to femoral artery pulsation.
  - Aim parallel to femoral pulse (toward umbilicus if no pulse); 30–45° angle to skin.
  - Vein should be entered within 5 cm.
  - If no pulse is palpable (e.g., cardiac arrest), the vein is approximately 2/3 the distance from the anterior superior iliac crest to the ipsilateral pubic tubercle; the pulse palpable with CPR is felt **at the femoral vein**, so aim for the palpated pulse.

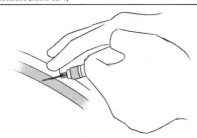

FIGURE 32-9. Femoral Vein Catheterization

The fingers are palpating the left femoral pulse and the introducer needle is advanced 1 cm medial to the femoral pulse at a 45° angle aiming toward the umbilicus.

COMPLICATIONS (TABLE 32-1)

TABLE 32-1. Complications of Central Venous Catheter Placement

Complication	Subclavian vein	Internal jugular vein	Femoral vein
Catheter-related blood stream infection (per 1000 line days)	4	8.6	15.3
Pneumothorax	1.5–3.1%	0.1–0.2%	N/A
Hemothorax	0.4–0.6%	< 0.1%	N/A
Catheter malposition	1.8–9.3% (7%)	1.8–14% (5%)	N/A
Line-related vein thrombosis (per 1000 catheter days)	0–13 (8)	1.2–3	8–34 (21)
Arterial puncture	0.5–3.1%	3.0–6.3%	6–9%
Hematoma	1.2–2.1%	0.1–2.2%	3.8–4.4%
Arrhythmia	Atrial dysrhythmias in 28–41%; ventricular ectopy in up to 25%		N/A
Cardiac perforation	Very rare		N/A
Air embolus	Negligible if performed in Trendelenberg position		
Lost guidewire	Negligible if operator maintains control of guidewire		

Source: Data from *NEJM*. 2007; 356: e21, *NEJM*. 2003; 348: 1123–1133, and *Ann Thoracic Med*. 2007; 2: 61–3.

CODING

36556	Introduction of non-tunnelled central venous catheter (> 5 years old)
36555	Introduction of non-tunnelled central venous catheter (< 5 years old)
36800	Dialysis catheter placement
36597	Reposition central venous catheter
76937	Ultrasound guidance for central lines

REFERENCES

NEJM. 2007; 356: e21.
Arch Int Med. 2004; 164: 842–850.
Arch Surg. 2004; 139: 131–136.
NEJM. 2003; 348: 1123–1133.
Crit Care Med. 2005; 33: 13.
BMJ. 2003; 327: 361.
JAMA. 2001; 286: 700.
Acad Emer Med. 2002; 9: 800.
Anesth. 2002; 97: 528.
Crit Care Med. 2007; 35S: S178–S185.
Ann Thoracic Med. 2007; 2: 61–63.

33 ■ ARTERIAL LINE PLACEMENT

INDICATIONS

- Management of shock states
- Continuous blood pressure monitoring
- Continuous cardiac output monitoring
- Frequent arterial blood gas sampling
- Consider if need for very frequent blood draws
  - Severe diabetic ketoacidosis
  - Severe hyponatremia
  - Severe hypernatremia

CONTRAINDICATIONS

- Insufficient collateral circulation from the ulnar artery
  - Assess collateral circulation with a modified Allen test
  - Modified Allen test
    - Compress ulnar and radial arteries with fist clenched
    - Raise clenched fist above patient's head for one minute
    - Lower arm, relax fist, release ulnar artery but continue radial artery compression
    - Normal perfusion should return within six seconds
- Severe Raynaud's syndrome
- Thromboangiitis obliterans (Buerger disease)
- Overlying cellulitis or full-thickness burns to area of insertion
- Major injury to the extremity
- Need for thrombolytic therapy
- Lymphatic obstruction in the extremity proximal to the cannulation site
- Presence of an arteriovenous shunt in the extremity (relative contra-indication)
- Bleeding diathesis (relative contraindication)
  - Coagulopathy (INR > 2 or PTT > 2× upper limit of normal)
  - Platelets < 50,000

EQUIPMENT

- 20-gauge radial artery catheter-over-wire kit or 20-gauge angiocatheter
- Pressure transducer tubing
- Pressure transducer

- 4-0 silk or nylon suture
- Armboard
- Tape
- 1% lidocaine for skin anesthesia
- Flexible guidewire (for femoral/brachial arterial lines)
- No. 11 scalpel (for femoral/brachial arterial lines)
- Sterile occlusive dressing

TECHNIQUE FOR RADIAL ARTERIAL LINE

- Informed consent.
- Perform a "time out" procedure to confirm correct patient, site, and procedure.
- Use an armboard with mild wrist extension for radial arterial line placement.
- Wash hands and then don sterile attire.
- Radial artery is palpated ~2 cm proximal the wrist crease (**Figure 33-1**).
- Use lidocaine **without epinephrine** around artery (minimizes arterial vasospasm).

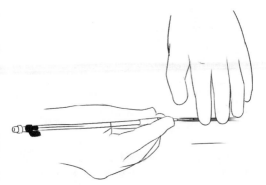

FIGURE 33-1. Radial Arterial Line Catheter Insertion

The radial artery pulse is palpated with two fingers to determine the optimal catheter insertion site and artery direction. An arterial line catheter is inserted just distal to the felt radial pulse at a 30° angle.

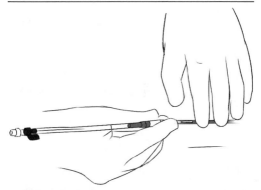

FIGURE 33-2. Arterial Flash Is Seen

The radial artery catheter is inserted until an arterial flash is seen within the catheter lumen. At this point, stop advancing the catheter and advance the wire through the needle.

- Take your time locating the maximal impulse.
  - Your first shot is your best shot.
- Advance needle at a 30–45° angle until arterial flash seen; then lower catheter angle to 10–15° (**Figure 33-2**).
  - Advance wire through needle (radial arterial line kit) (see **Figure 33-3** and **Figure 33-4**) or catheter over needle (angiocatheter).
- Advance catheter over wire if using a radial arterial line kit (**Figure 33-5**).
- Remove wire and needle, leaving catheter in place.
- Attach pressure transducer tubing to catheter hub and assure that a good arterial waveform is seen on the monitor (**Figure 33-6**).
- Secure catheter in place with suture.
- Place a clear, sterile occlusive dressing over insertion site.

TECHNIQUE FOR FEMORAL OR BRACHIAL ARTERIAL LINES

- Consider using an ultrasound for brachial artery or femoral arterial line placement.
  - Real-time ultrasound guidance requires a sterile sheath and sterile ultrasound gel.

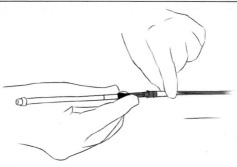

FIGURE 33-3. Wire Threaded Through Arterial Catheter Needle

Once an arterial flash is seen, the catheter is held steady as the wire is advanced fully through the needle into the artery.

- Brachial artery typically cannulated about 5 cm above the elbow.
- Femoral artery typically cannulated 2–3 cm below the inguinal crease.
- Modified Seldinger technique utilized to place brachial or femoral arterial lines:
  - Introducer needle is used to cannulate the artery at a 30–45° angle.
  - Syringe is detached from the needle and pulsatile blood is confirmed.
  - Thread guidewire through the needle.

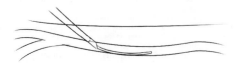

FIGURE 33-4. Wire Threaded Through Arterial Catheter and Needle
Adapted from Custalow CB. *Color Atlas of Emergency Department Procedures.* Philadelphia, PA: Saunders; 2004: 131, Figure 4.

Cross section of the artery demonstrating how the wire is advanced through the needle and into the artery.

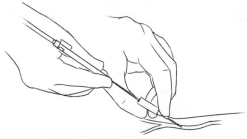

FIGURE 33-5. Advancing a Radial Catheter Over Wire
Adapted from Custalow CB. *Color Atlas of Emergency Department Procedures.* Philadelphia, PA: Saunders; 2004: 132, Figure 5.

After the wire has been advanced, the catheter kit is held steady as the white catheter is advanced with a twisting motion until the catheter hub is at the skin. The needle and the wire are then withdrawn, leaving the arterial catheter in place.

- Withdraw the needle, leaving the wire in place.
- Use a scalpel to nick the skin over the wire.
- Advance the catheter over the wire until the hub is at the skin; then withdraw the wire.
- Attach pressure transducer tubing to catheter hub and assure that a good arterial waveform is seen on the monitor.

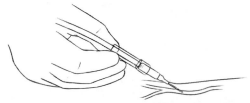

FIGURE 33-6. Connecting Arterial Catheter to Pressure Transducer Tubing

Once the arterial catheter is in place, pressure transducer tubing is screwed onto the catheter hub and an arterial waveform should be seen on the monitor screen.

- Secure catheters in place with suture.
- Place a clear, sterile occlusive dressing over insertion site.

COMPLICATIONS

- **Major Complications**
  - Arterial thrombosis (< 1%)
  - Catheter embolization (very rare)
  - Pseudoaneurysm (especially in femoral location, very rare)
  - Arteriovenous fistula (especially in femoral location, very rare)
- **Minor Complications**
  - Catheter-related bloodstream infection (0.5%)
  - Bleeding (2%)
  - Hematoma
  - Median nerve impairment (especially with prolonged wrist hyperextension)

CODING

36620   Percutaneous arterial line placement

76937   Vascular ultrasound

REFERENCES

NEJM. 2006; 354: e13–e14.
Roberts JR, Hedges JR, eds. *Clinical Procedures in Emergency Medicine.* 5th ed. Philadelphia, PA: Saunders; 2009: 349–363.
Chen H, Sonnenday CJ, eds. *Manual of Common Bedside Surgical Procedures.* 2nd ed. Philadelphia, PA: Lippincott Williams & Wilkins; 2000: 69–80.
Anesthesiology, 2004; 100: 287–291.

34 ■ PULMONARY ARTERY CATHETER INSERTION

INDICATIONS

- Assessment and management of shock states
- Management of refractory pulmonary edema (cardiogenic vs ARDS)
- Hemodynamically unstable patients refractory to conventional therapy
- Optimization of cardiac index in cardiogenic shock
- Optimization of therapy in refractory heart failure
- Preoperative optimization of extremely high-risk surgical patients
- Need for pacing using a temporary pacing pulmonary artery catheter
- Evaluation and drug titration for severe pulmonary hypertension
- Diagnostic evaluation of left-to-right cardiac shunts
- Pretransplantation workup

ABSOLUTE CONTRAINDICATIONS

- Presence of a right ventricular assist device
- Prosthetic right heart valve
- Transvenous pacemaker or defibrillator
- Right ventricular mural thrombus or mass
- Latex allergy
- Infection or full-thickness burn at the insertion site

RELATIVE CONTRAINDICATIONS

- Severe coagulopathy
  - PTT > 1.5 × upper limit of normal
  - INR > 1.5 in patient on warfarin
- Thrombocytenia (platelets < 50K)
- Left bundle branch block (0.1–5% risk of complete heart block)
- Right-sided endocarditis without vegetation by echocardiogram
- Uncontrolled ventricular or atrial dysrhythmias
- Prior pneumonectomy

EQUIPMENT

- 9 French percutaneous sheath introducer kit (Cordis catheter kit)
- Chlorhexidine or povidone-iodine swabs
- 8 French radiopaque pulmonary artery catheter (PAC) kit (**Figure 34-1**)

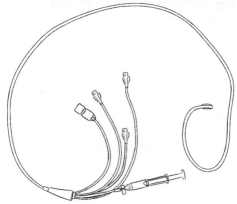

FIGURE 34-1. Pulmonary Artery Catheter

The pulmonary artery catheter has a natural curve at the end of the catheter.

- Pressure transducer and high-pressure tubing, connectors and two three-way stopcocks
- Cardiac monitor
- Heparinized lines for three catheter ports
- Sterile gown and gloves
- Face mask
- Surgical cap

TECHNIQUE

- Informed consent by patient or surrogate decision-maker, if possible.
- Perform "time out" procedure to confirm the correct patient, procedure, and location of procedure.
- Place patient on a cardiac monitor.
- Wash hands and then don sterile attire.
- Sterile prep of skin with chlorhexidine.
- Wide sterile drape of area.

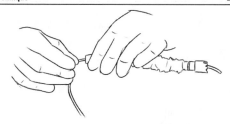

FIGURE 34-2. Sterile Sheath Placed Over Pulmonary Artery Catheter

A sterile sheath is inserted over the pulmonary artery catheter and secured in place at the 100-cm mark on the catheter.

- Introduce a 9 French percutaneous introducer sheath (Cordis catheter) using Modified Seldinger technique.
  - Best locations for PAC placement are the right internal jugular vein or the left subclavian vein
- Place a sterile sheath over the PAC and secure it in place at the 100-cm mark of the catheter (**Figure 34-2**).
  - Assure that the locking adapter of the sheath is facing the tip of the PAC.
- Flush each port of the catheter with sterile saline.
- The "CVP" and "PA" ports of the catheter are than connected to pressure transducer tubing.
- Calibrate and zero the equipment and level the pressure transducer.
- Inflate the balloon with 1.5 ml air and assure that it inflates properly (**Figure 34-3**).
- Wiggle the tip of the PAC and the catheter waveform on the monitor should respond.
- Introduce the PAC into the Cordis catheter hub with the curve of the PAC directed toward the heart (**Figure 34-4**).
- Advance the catheter with the balloon deflated about 15 cm.
- Inflate the balloon and the waveform should be a central venous or right atrial tracing.
- Advance the PAC fairly quickly with the balloon inflated, and the waveform should change to a right ventricular waveform, then a pulmonary artery waveform.
- Once a pulmonary artery waveform is seen, advance the PAC slowly until a pulmonary capillary wedge pressure tracing is seen; usually 45–55 cm from the internal jugular or subclavian vein insertion sites (**Figure 34-5**).

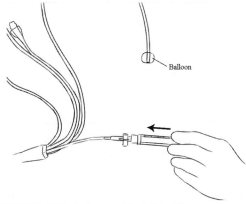

FIGURE 34-3. Testing the Pulmonary Artery Catheter Balloon

The pulmonary artery catheter (PAC) balloon is inflated with 1.5 ml air. Its integrity is always tested prior to insertion of the PAC.

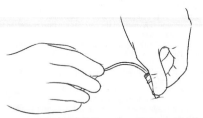

FIGURE 34-4. Inserting the Pulmonary Artery Catheter Through the Introducer Sheath

The pulmonary artery catheter is inserted through an introducer sheath that has previously been inserted into a central vein. The curve of the pulmonary artery catheter is directed inferiorly for a subclavian vein placement and directed toward the patient's left for an internal jugular vein placement.

Pulmonary Artery Catheter Waveforms Configurations During Insertion

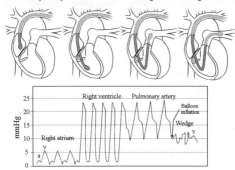

FIGURE 34-5. Pulmonary Artery Catheter Waveforms Configurations During Insertion

Adapted from Ashworth K, Hayes M. Bedside Pulmonary Arterial Catheterization. In: Fink M, Abraham E, Vincent J-L, et al., eds. *Textbook of Critical Care.* 5th ed. Philadelphia, PA: Saunders; 2005: 1802, Figure 209-1.

- At this point, a deflated balloon will show the pulmonary artery waveform and an inflated balloon will show a pulmonary capillary wedge pressure tracing.
- Lock the sheath in place (**Figure 34-6**).
- Apply a sterile, occlusive dressing over the insertion site.

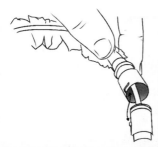

FIGURE 34-6. Closing the Sterile Sheath Over the Pulmonary Artery Catheter

Once the pulmonary artery catheter has been fully inserted, the sterile sheath is locked in place onto the percutaneous sheath.

- Obtain a CXR to confirm proper PAC tip placement.
- The pulmonary capillary wedge pressure should be measured at end-expiration.
- Flush catheter lines with heparinized saline every 30–60 minutes.

COMPLICATIONS

- Complications from cordis catheter placement
  - Pneumothorax
  - Arterial puncture
  - Air embolus
  - Venous thrombosis
- Atrial or ventricular dysrhythmias
- Right bundle branch block (0.1–5% of insertions)
- Pulmonary infarction
- Pulmonary artery rupture (0.2% incidence)
  - Inflate balloon to tamponade vessel and obtain a stat cardiothoracic surgery consult.
- Catheter-related bloodstream infection
- Marantic or infectious endocarditis
- Mural thrombus
- Knotting of catheter
- Cardiac perforation and tamponade (extremely rare)
- Balloon rupture

CODING

93503   Insertion and placement of a flow-directed catheter for monitoring purposes

76937   Ultrasound guidance for venous cannulation

REFERENCES

Crit Care Med. 2005; 33: 1119–1122.
Crit Care Med. 2004; 32: 691–699.
JAMA. 2005; 294: 1693–1694.
N Engl J Med. 2001; 345: 1368–1377.
Lung. 2005; 183: 209–219.
Circulation. 2009; 119: 147–152.
Cochrane Database Syst Rev 3. 2006; CD003408.
JAMA. 2007; 298: 458–461.
JAMA. 2005; 294: 1664–1670.

35 ■ INTRAOSSEOUS LINE PLACEMENT

- Emergency vascular access in children or adults
- May administer all ACLS medications, vasopressors, anesthetic agents, antitoxins
- Capable of rapid infusions of crystalloid or colloid solutions, including blood products

CONTRAINDICATIONS

- Osteogenesis imperfecta
- Severe osteoporosis (relative)
- Ipsilateral fracture or crush injury
- Extremity with a vascular injury
- Full-thickness burn or infection at insertion site

EQUIPMENT

- Sterile gloves
- Sterile gown
- Facemask with shield
- Sterile fenestrated drape
- Bone marrow aspirate needle (e.g., Illinois or Jamshidi aspirate needles) or an intraosseous needle (e.g., Cook modified Dieckmann needle) **(Figure 35-1)**
- Antiseptic solution: chlorhexidine or povidone-iodine swabs
- 2% lidocaine
- 5-ml syringe

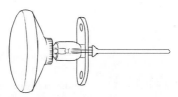

FIGURE 35-1. Intraosseous Needle

- 10-ml Luer-lok syringe
- IV tubing
- Sterile 4 × 4-inch gauze
- Tape
- Rolled towel

TECHNIQUE

- Identify the insertion site (see **Figure 35-2**).
- Place a rolled towel under the knee for a proximal tibial intraosseous line placement.
- Using antiseptic solution to prep skin.
- In alert patients, anesthetize skin and periosteum at insertion site with 1% lidocaine.
- Grasp the intraosseous needle and stabilize the shaft between the index and middle finger of the dominant hand.
- Insert the needle through the skin and perpendicular to the bone (**Figure 35-2**).
- Advance needle through the bone with a twisting motion until the cortex is penetrated, at which point a loss of resistance will be felt and the needle will no longer rock back and forth.
- Remove the inner stylet and attach a 10-ml syringe to the needle hub (**Figure 35-3**).
- Aspirate marrow to confirm intramedullary placement of the needle (**Figure 35-4**).
- In conscious patients, for anesthesia, in children flush needle with 1 mg/kg of 2% lidocaine (20 mg/ml) as a slow IV push; in adults use 2.5 ml 2% lidocaine slow IV push.
- Flush needle with 5 ml sterile saline to guarantee a lack of resistance to flow.

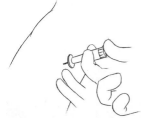

FIGURE 35-2. Advancing Intraosseous Needle Through Bony Cortex

The intraosseous needle is inserted into the medial aspect of the proximal tibia with a rotating motion.

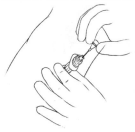

FIGURE 35-3. Removing Cap and Stylet from the Intraosseous Needle

The intraosseous needle is advanced through the bony cortex until a loss of resistance is felt, at which point the needle should not wobble. The cap and stylet and then removed from the needle.

- Remove the syringe and connect the IV tubing to the needle (**Figure 35-5**).
- Begin IV fluid and medication administration.
- Surround needle with sterile gauze and tape in place.
- Ideally, the intraosseous needle should be removed within 24 hours, but it may be left in place for up to 72 hours if necessary.
- To remove needle, screw a 10-ml Luer-Lok syringe onto the needle and then rotate the syringe clockwise as traction is pulled.

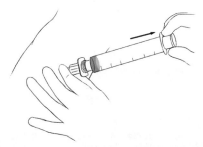

FIGURE 35-4. Aspiration of Bone Marrow Through Intraosseous Needle

A 10-ml syringe is attached to the needle and then bone marrow is aspirated to confirm proper location of the needle.

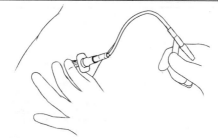

FIGURE 35-5. Connecting IV Tubing to Intraosseous Needle

Once the placement of the intraosseous needle is confirmed, IV tubing is attached to the needle hub.

COMPLICATIONS

- Needle insertion through entire bone
- Extravasation of fluid into soft tissue
  - May cause tissue necrosis if vasopressors extravasate
  - May cause compartment syndrome
- Infection (soft tissue or osteomyelitis)
- Bone fracture (especially if severe osteoporosis)
- Growth plate disruption
- Fat embolism (very rare)

CODING

36680   Placement of needle for intraosseous infusion

REFERENCES

Emerg Med Serv. 2005; 34: 54.

J Emerg Med. 1989; 7: 587.

Roberts JR, Hedges JR, eds. *Clinical Procedures in Emergency Medicine.* 5th ed. Philadelphia, PA: Saunders; 2009: 431–442.

Ann Emerg Med. 1985; 14 (9): 885–888.

J Emerg Med. 2010; 39 (4): 468–475.

INDEX

Note: Italicized page locators indicate a figure; tables are noted with a *t.*

A

ABG. *See* Arterial blood gas
Abscesses, incision and
  drainage of, 69–72
  anesthesia for, *70*
  blunt dissection to break
    up loculations
    within abscess
    cavity, *71*
  coding, 72
  complications, 72
  contraindications, 69
  equipment, 69
  indications, 69
  packing abscess cavity, *71*
  references, 72
  scalpel incision of
    abscess wall, *70*
  technique, 69–71
Acrocordon, 46
Actinic keratoses, 46
Acute Respiratory Distress
    Syndrome,
    noninvasive
    positive-pressure
    ventilation and,
    19, 22
Adaptic, 44
Adenosine deaminase
    level, CSF studies
    and, 138
Adson forceps, skin lesion
    excised with, *57*
Adults
  medications for
    procedural sedation
    in, 6*t*–7*t*
  options for moderate-
    deep sedation in, 8
AFB RNA by PCR, CSF
    studies and, 138
Air leaks, chest tubes
    and, 184
Airway assessment, for
    potentially difficult
    oral intubation, 3, *5*

Airway procedures, 10–23
  endotracheal intubation,
    11–18
  noninvasive positive-
    pressure
    ventilation, 19–23
Albumin, paracentesis and, 89
Allen test, modified, 197
Allis clamp, excision
    technique for
    large lipomas/
    subcutaneous
    masses and, 75, *76*
Aluminum chloride, shave
    skin biopsy and, 51
Anemia, unexplained, bone
    marrow aspiration/
    biopsy and, 127
Angiotensin converting
    enzyme (ACE)
    levels, CSF studies
    and, 138
Ankylosing spondylitis,
    endotracheal
    intubation and, 11
Anterior epistaxis, 81
  dual balloon nasal
    catheters and, *84*
  selecting options for, 82
Anterior-posterior pads,
    placing for
    transcutaneous
    pacing, *36*
Anterior superior iliac
    spine, biopsy sites
    for, 128
Anterior tibia, biopsy sites
    for, 128
Anterolateral pads, placing
    for transcutaneous
    pacing, *36*
Antibiotics
  incision/drainage of
    abscesses and
    indications for, 71
  laceration repair and, 44

Antipsychotics, mechanical
    ventilation
    and, 175
APACHE II score, NPPV
    and, 22
ARDS. *See* Acute respiratory
    distress syndrome
Arm casts, 148–149
  long, *149*
  short, *148*
  thumb spica cast, *148*
Arm splints, *147–148*
  posterior long arm
    splint, *148*
  sugar tong splint, *147*
  ulnar gutter splint, *147*
  volar short arm
    splint, *147*
Arterial blood gas, NPPV
    monitoring
    and, 22
Arterial line placement,
    197–202
  coding, 202
  complications, major and
    minor, 202
  contraindications, 197
  equipment, 197–198
  femoral or brachial
    arterial lines,
    technique for,
    199–202
  indications, 197
  radial arterial line,
    technique for,
    198–199
  references, 202
Arthrocentesis, 153–158
  absolute contraindications,
    153
  coding, 158
  complications, 158
  diagnostic, indications,
    153
  elbow, technique,
    156–158

Arthrocentesis—*Continued*
equipment, 153–154
knee, technique, 154–155
references, 158
relative
contraindications,
153
shoulder, technique,
155–156
synovial fluid analysis,
158
therapeutic, indications,
153
Ascitic fluid
analysis of, 91, 92t
aspiration of, 90
classification of, 91t
Assist control (AC),
mechanical
ventilation, 175
Atrial fibrillation,
synchronized
cardioversion and
initial energy levels
for, 33t
Atrial flutter, synchronized
cardioversion and
initial energy levels
for, 33t
Atropine, rapid sequence
intubation and, 13

B

Bacterial meningitis,
predictors of, 139
Balloon catheter, in place,
for epistaxis, 84
Basal cell carcinomas,
shave skin biopsy
and, 50
Bayonet forceps, intranasal
device placement
for epistaxis and,
81, 82
Benzodiazepines,
mechanical
ventilation and,
175
Betamethasone, for joint
injections, 160t
Bilevel positive airway
pressure (BiPAP)
preparing patient for, 21
strapped in place, 21

technique for, 20,
20–21, 21
Biopsies. See Bone marrow
aspiration and
biopsy; Endometrial
biopsy; Skin
biopsies
BiPAP. See Bilevel positive
airway pressure
Bone marrow aspirate
needle, introducing,
129
Bone marrow aspiration and
biopsy, 127–133
biopsy sites, 128
bone marrow aspirate
optional studies,
133
coding, 133
complications, 133
contraindications, 127
equipment, 127–128
indications, 127
obtaining bone marrow
aspirate, 130
references, 133
technique
for posterior superior
iliac spine bone
marrow aspirate,
129–130
for posterior superior
iliac spine bone
marrow core biopsy,
130–133
Bowen's disease, 46
Brachial artery, cannulating,
200
Broom device, endocervix
and ectocervix
sampled with,
111, 111
Buerger disease, 197
BURP maneuver,
endotracheal
intubation and, 14

C

Cardiac procedures, 24–37
pericardiocentesis,
25–30
synchronized
cardioversion,
31–34

transcutaneous pacing,
35–37
Cardiac tamponade, causes
of, in U.S., 25
Cardioversion, paddles used
for, in anterolateral
position, 33
Casting extremities
application of cast
material over Webril
for, 145
arm casts, 148–149
basic technique for,
144–151
coding, 151–152
complications, 151
contraindications, 141
equipment, 141
folding Webril and
stockinette over
cast material, 145
indications, 141
leg casts, 150–151
molding cast into proper
position, 146
postprocedure care, 151
references, 152
rolling cast material
over Webril and
stockinette, 146
Cast material, applying for
splinting, 143, 143
Central venous access,
187–196
cannulating vein, 189
central venous catheter
introduced over
wire, 191
coding, 196
complications, 195t
contraindications for
central venous
catheter placement,
187
dilating the skin and
subcutaneous tissue
over the wire, 190
equipment, 187–188
femoral vein catheters,
194, 195
general technique
for central line
placement for all
locations, 188

indications for central venous catheters, 187
internal jugular vein catheters, 192–193
central approach, *192*, 192–193
posterior approach, 193
nicking skin with scalpel over the wire, *190*
references, 196
securing central venous catheter in place, *191*
subclavian vein catheters, 193
infraclavicular approach, 193, *194*
supraclavicular approach, 193
threading wire through introducer needle, *189*

Central venous catheter introducing over wire, *191*
securing in place, *191*

Cervix, visualizing, 109

Cherry angiomas, 46

Chest tube
inserting, *183*
placement
blunt dissection during, *183*
local anesthesia for, *181*
proper positioning for, *181*
skin incision for, *182*
securing with suture, *184*

Children, anxiolysis in, 8

Chin length, endotracheal intubation and, 11

Chloral hydrate, anxiolysis in children and, 8

Chromic sutures, excision technique for large lipomas/subcutaneous masses and, 76

Chylothorax, tube thoracostomy and, 179

Circumcision with Gomco clamp, 101–107
applying Gomco bell, 104
clearing adhesions between foreskin and glans, *102*
coding, 106
complications, 106
contraindications, 101
creating dorsal foreskin crush, *103*
creating dorsal slit, *103*
elevating foreskin through base plate, *105*
equipment, 101
excising foreskin, *106*
indications, 101
postprocedure care, 105–106
references, 107
technique, 102–105

Clubfoot deformities, casting for, 141

Cocci titer, CSF studies and, 138

Coding
abscesses, incision and drainage of, 72
arterial line placement, 202
arthrocentesis, 158
bone marrow aspiration and biopsy, 133
central venous access, 196
cryosurgery of skin lesions, 48–49
endometrial biopsy, 117
endotracheal intubation, 18
epistaxis, intranasal device placement for, 85
excisional skin biopsy, 58
ingrown toenails removal, 68
intraosseous line placement, 212
intrauterine device insertion, 124
removal, 125
joint injections, 163
for laceration repair, 45*t*

lipoma or subcutaneous mass excision, 77
lumbar puncture, 139
mechanical ventilation, 178
newborn circumcision with Gomco clamp, 106
for noninvasive positive-pressure ventilation, 23
Pap smear, 113
paracentesis, 92
pericardiocentesis, 30
procedural sedation, 8
pulmonary artery catheter insertion, 208
punch skin biopsy, 60
shave skin biopsy, 52
spirometry, 168
splinting and casting of extremities, 151–152
synchronized cardioversion, 34
thoracentesis, 174
transcutaneous pacing, 37
tube thoracostomy, 185
tympanometry, 37
vasectomy, no-scalpel, 100

Colposcopy, 113

Continuous positive airway pressure, 20, 22

Cook modified Dieckmann needle, 209

Cordis catheter kit, pulmonary artery catheter insertion and, 203, 205

Cordis catheter placement, complications, 208

Corticosteroids, for joint injections, 160*t*

Cotton pledgets
intranasal device placement for epistaxis and, 81, *82*
placement of, into nasal cavity, *83*

CPAP. *See* Continuous positive airway pressure

CPT codes, for laceration
  repair, 45t
Cryoprobe, technique, 46, 47
Cryosurgery of skin lesions,
    46–49
  coding, 48–49
  complications, 48
  contraindications, 46
  equipment, 46
  ice ball creation, 48
  indications, 46
  postprocedure care, 48
  references, 49
  technique for liquid
      nitrogen spray
      gun or cryoprobe,
      46–47, 47
  technique for Q-tip
      application, 47
Cryptococcal antigen, CSF
  studies and, 138
CSF (cerebrospinal fluid)
  collecting in sterile
      collection tubes, 138
  normal values in adults,
      138t
  routine and optional
      studies of, 138
CT scan of head, obtaining
  prior to lumbar
  puncture, 138
Cytobrush
  rolling across slide,
      111, 111
  sampling endocervical
      canal with, 109,
      110
Cytogenetic analysis, 133

D

"Deadly triangles,"
  excisional skin
  biopsy and, 53–54
Deep interrupted suture,
  with buried knot, 41
Defasciculating agent,
  rapid sequence
  intubation and, 13
Dermabond, 40
Dermatology, 38–77
  cryosurgery of skin
      lesions, 46–49
  excisional skin biopsy,
      53–58

incision and drainage of
  abscesses, 69–72
ingrown toenails removal,
  63–68
laceration repair, 39–45
lipoma or subcutaneous
  mass excision,
  73–77
punch skin biopsy, 59–62
shave skin biopsy, 50–52
Dexmedetomidine,
  mechanical
  ventilation and,
  175
Dexon, 40
Diazepam, vasectomy
  premedication
  with, 95
Digital nerve block, ingrown
  toenails removal
  and, 64, 64
Dorsal foreskin crush,
  creating, 103
Down Syndrome,
  endotracheal
  intubation and, 12
Dressings, for laceration
  repair, 44
Dressler's syndrome, 25
Dual-balloon catheters
  inflated, in place, 85
  nasal, for epistaxis,
  84, 84
Dyspnea, unexplained,
  spirometry and, 165

E

Ear, nose, and throat
  procedures, 78–85
  intranasal device
      placement for
      epistaxis, 81–85
  tympanometry, 79–80
Ectocervix
  sampling with broom
      device, 111, 111
  sampling with spatula,
      109, 110
Elastic wrap, wrapping over
  cast material for
  splinting, 144
Elbow arthrocentesis
  technique for, 156–158
  landmarks for, 157

Encephalitis panel, CSF
  studies and, 138
Endocell, endometrial biopsy
  and, 114
Endocervical canal,
  sampling with
  cytobrush, 109, 110
Endocervix, sampling with
  broom device, 109,
  110
Endometrial aspirator,
  inserting, 115
Endometrial biopsy,
    114–117
  coding, 117
  complications, 117
  contraindications, 114
  endometrial sampling,
      116
  equipment, 114
  indications, 114
  insertion of endometrial
      aspirator, 115
  postprocedure care, 117
  references, 117
  sample expelled into
      formalin jar, 117
  technique, 114–117
  withdrawal of internal
      piston, 116
Endometrial dating, 114
Endotracheal intubation,
    11–18
  airway assessment, 11
  coding, 18
  common induction
      agents, 16–17
  common paralytic
      agents, 17–18
  complications, 18
  equipment, 12–13
  indications, 11
  inflating endotracheal
      tube cuff, 16
  insertion of endotracheal
      tube, 15
  Macintosh blade
      introduced for direct
      laryngoscopy, 15
  morbidly obese patients
      and "ramp"
      position for, 14
  predictors of difficult
      airway, 11–12

exam features, 12
history, 11–12
preparation for, 12
proper sniffing position
for, *13*
references, 18
seven Ps of rapid
sequence
intubation,
13–14, 16
special considerations
for, 11
Endotracheal tube
inserting, *15*
securing, *17*
End-tidal carbon dioxide
monitors, ventilator
weaning and, 175
Enucleation technique, for
small lipomas, 74
ePAP
biPAP technique and, 20
machine settings, 21
Epi-Max Balloon Catheter, 84
Epistat catheter, 84
Epistaxis, intranasal device
placement for,
81–85
balloon catheter in
place, *84*
coding, 85
complications, 84–85
contraindications, 81
cotton pledget and, *82*
dual balloon nasal
catheters, *84*
equipment, 81
indications, 81
inflated dual-balloon
catheter in position,
85
placement of cotton
pledgets into nasal
cavity, *83*
placement of Merocel
tampons, *83*
references, 85
technique, 82–84
Epi-Stop Balloon Catheter,
anterior epistaxis
and, 82
Eschmann stylet,
endotracheal tube
and, 16

Etomidate
endotracheal intubation
and, 16
moderate-deep sedation
in adults and, 8
procedural sedation in
adults and, *7t*
synchronized
cardioversion
and, 32
Eustachian tube
dysfunction,
tympanometry and
evaluation of, 79
Excisional skin biopsy,
53–58
coding, 58
complications, 58
contraindications, 53
elliptical incision
around, *57*
equipment, 53
excising skin lesion, *57*
indications, 53
Lines of Langer
body, *55*
face, *56*
postprocedure care, 58
references, 58
technique, 53–54
Exudates, causes of, 173

F
Face mask
determining size of,
20, *20*
patient intolerance of, 22
FACTS check, splinting of
extremities and,
144
Femoral arterial line,
technique for,
199–202
Femoral artery, cannulating,
200
Femoral vein catheters,
194, *195*
Fentanyl
mechanical ventilation
and, 175
moderate-deep sedation
in adults and, 8
procedural sedation in
adults and, *6t*

rapid sequence
intubation and, 13
synchronized
cardioversion
and, 32
FEV$_1$, in obstructive lung
disease, 167, *168t*
Fiberoptic oral intubation, 11
FISH analysis, molecular
cytogenetics
by, 133
Flow volume curves,
spirograms and, *167*
Foreskin
creating dorsal slit, *103*
elevating through base
plate, *105*
excising, *106*
hemostat used to break
up adhesions
under, *102*
Frova stylet, endotracheal
tube and, 16
FVC, restrictive lung disease
and interpretation
of, 167, *168t*

G
Gastrointestinal procedures,
paracentesis,
87–93
Gene rearrangement
studies, by
polymerase chain
reaction, 133
Genitourinary procedures,
94–107
newborn circumcision
with Gomco clamp,
101–107
no-scalpel vasectomy,
95–100
Glenohumeral joint injection
corticosteroids for, *160t*
technique, 160
Gomco bell
applying over glans,
104, *104*
excising foreskin around,
106
hemostat used to
reapproximate
dorsal slit around,
104

Gomco clamp, newborn circumcision with, 101–107, *104, 105, 106*

Greater trochanteric bursa, corticosteroids for, 160*t*

Guillain-Barré syndrome, diagnostic lumbar puncture and, 135

Gynecologic procedures, 108–125
endometrial biopsy, 114–117
intrauterine device insertion/removal, 118–125
Pap smear, 109–113

H

Hearing impairment, tympanometry and evaluation of, 79

Hematology/oncology procedures, 126–133
bone marrow aspiration and biopsy, 127–133

Hemostat
for breaking up loculations within abscess cavity, 71, *71*
ingrown toenails removal and, *66*

Hemothorax, tube thoracostomy and, 179

Horizontal mattress suture, 40, *43*

HPV DNA testing, Pap smear and, 113

Hypercapnia, unexplained, spirometry and, 165

Hypoxia, unexplained, spirometry and, 165

I

Ice ball, cryosurgery and creation of, 46, 47, *48*

Illinois aspirate needle, 209

India ink study, CSF studies and, 138

Induction agents, endotracheal intubation and, 16–17

Informed consent
central venous access and, 188
paracentesis and, 88
posterior superior iliac spine bone marrow aspirate and, 129
pulmonary artery catheter insertion and, 204
radial arterial line placement and, 198
thoracentesis and, 170
tube thoracostomy and, 180

Infraclavicular approach, to subclavian vein catheterization, 193, *194*

Ingrown toenails removal, 63–68
coding, 68
complications, 67
contraindications, 63
cutting affected area of nail, *65*
digital block of toe, *64*
equipment, 63
indications, 63
nail ablation with phenol, *67*
postprocedure care, 67
references, 68
removal of inflamed granulation tissue, *66*
removing affected area of nail, *66*
separation of nail from nail matrix, *65*
technique, 64, *65, 66, 67,* 67

Internal jugular vein catheterization
central approach to, *192,* 192–193
posterior approach to, 193

Interrupted nylon sutures, excision technique

for large lipomas/subcutaneous masses and, 76

Intranasal device placement for epistaxis, 81–85

Intraosseous line placement, 209–212
coding, 212
complications, 212
contraindications, 209
equipment, 209–210
indications, 209
references, 212
technique, 210–211

Intraosseous needle, *209*
advancing through bony cortex, *210*
aspiration of bone marrow through, *211*
IV line connected to, *212*
removing cap and stylet from, *211*

Intrauterine device
insertion, 118–125
coding, 124
complications, 124
contraindications, 118
equipment, 118
indications, 118
technique for Mirena IUD insertion, 121–123
technique for Paragard T380A insertion, 119–120
references, 125
removal
coding, 125
complications, 125
contraindications, 124
equipment, 124
indications, 124
postprocedure care, 125
technique, 124–125

Intubation. *See* Endotracheal intubation

iPAP
BiPAP technique and, 20
machine settings, 21

Iris scissors, excision technique for large lipomas/subcutaneous masses and, 76

J

Jamshidi aspirate needle, 209
Jamshidi biopsy needle, 130
  advancing into bone marrow, *132*
  advancing through bony cortex, *131*
  pushing biopsy specimen out of, *132*
  removing stylet from, *131*
Jamshidi bone marrow aspiration and biopsy kit, 127
Jaw opening, endotracheal intubation and, 11
Joint injections, 159–163
  coding, 163
  complications, 163
  contraindications, 159
  corticosteroids for, 160*t*
  equipment, 159
  general technique for, 159–160
  glenohumeral joint injections, technique, 160
  indications, 159
  knee injection, technique, 160
  lateral epicondyle injection, technique, 161–162
  post-procedure care, 163
  references, 163
  subacromial bursa injection, technique, 160–161
  trochanteric bursa injection, technique, 163

K

Kelly clamp, chest tube placement and, 182, *183*

Keloids, 46
Ketamine
  endotracheal intubation and, 17
  mechanical ventilation and, 175
  procedural sedation in adults and, 6*t*
Ketofol
  moderate-deep sedation in adults and, 8
  procedural sedation in adults and, 7*t*
Knee arthrocentesis, technique, *154*, 154–155
Knee injection, technique, 160
Knee joint, corticosteroids for, 160*t*

L

Laceration repair, 39–45
  coding, 45*t*
  complications, 44
  contraindications, 39
  equipment, 39
  indications, 39
  postprocedure care, 44
  references, 45
  technique, 40, *41*, *42*, *43*, 44
Lactate study, CSF studies and, 138
Laryngoscope blade, endotracheal intubation and, 14
Laryngoscopy, direct, introduction of Macintosh blade for, *15*
Lateral epicondyle injection
  corticosteroids for, 160*t*
  technique for, 161–162, *162*
Leg casts, *150–151*
  long, *151*
  short, *150*
Leg splints, *149–150*
  posterior leg and stirrup splints, *150*
  posterior leg splint, *149*
Lesions, freeze times for, 47

Leukopenia, unexplained, bone marrow aspiration/biopsy and, 127
Lidocaine
  injection of, directly over vas, *97*
  paravasal injection of, after 2.5 cm advancement of needle in cephalic direction, *97*
  rapid sequence intubation and, 13
Lines of Langer
  body, *55*
  defined, 54
  face, *56*
  incision/drainage of abscesses and, 70
Lipoma or subcutaneous mass excision, 73–77
  coding, 77
  complications, 73
  contraindications, 73
  enucleation technique for small lipomas, 74–75
  equipment, 73–74
  expressing lipoma through skin incision, *75*
  indications, 73
  initial elliptical incision over lipoma, *76*
  large lipomas/subcutaneous masses, excision technique for, 75–76
  linear excision over lipoma, *74*
  lysing adhesions around lipoma, *74*
  references, 77
  sharp dissection around sides of lipoma, *76*
Liquid-based Pap testing, 112, 112*t*
Liquid nitrogen spray gun, technique, 46, *47*

LOAD mnemonic, rapid sequence intubation, 13

Long arm cast, *149*

Long leg cast, *151*

Lorazepam
anxiolysis in adults and, 5
mechanical ventilation and, 175
procedural sedation in adults and, 6*t*

Lumbar puncture, 135–139
coding, 139
collecting CSF in sterile collection tubes, *138*
complications, major and minor, 139
contraindications, 135
CSF studies, 138
equipment, 135–136
indications
diagnostic lumbar puncture, 135
therapeutic lumbar puncture, 135
insertion of spinal needle in the L3-4 interspace, *137*
predictors of bacterial meningitis, 139
references, 139
stylet removed from spinal needle, *137*
technique, 136–138
when to obtain CT scan of head prior to lumbar puncture, 138–139

Lung protective ventilation
indications, 175
PEEP-FiO2 algorithm for, 176*t*

M

Macintosh blade
endotracheal intubation and, 14
introduction of, for direct laryngoscopy, *15*

Mallampati Class
airway assessment for potentially difficult oral intubation, 3, *5*

determining, endotracheal intubation and, 11

Manometer, attachment of, to spinal needle, *137*

Mask fitting wheel, for determining optimal face mask size, 20, *20*

Mechanical ventilation, 175–177
choosing mode of, 175
coding, 178
complications, 176
general guidelines, 176
initiating, 175
monitoring during, 175
oxygenation settings, 175
references, 178
settings for, 175
weaning and liberation from, *177*

Meningitis, diagnostic lumbar puncture and, 135

Merocel Doyle nasal pack, anterior epistaxis and, 82

Merocel tampons
nasal, anterior epistaxis and, 82
placement of, *83*

Metzenbaum scissors, excision technique for large lipomas/ subcutaneous masses and, 75, *76*

Methylprednisolone, for joint injections, 160*t*

Midazolam
anxiolysis in adults and, 5
anxiolysis in children and, 8
endotracheal intubation and, 17
mechanical ventilation and, 175
procedural sedation in adults and, 6*t*
synchronized cardioversion and, 32

Miller blade, endotracheal intubation and, 14

Mirena IUD
insertion, *122*
adverse reactions, 124
deploying, *123*
equipment, 118
indications, 118
loading, *122*
preparing, *121*
releasing, *123*
technique, 121
replacement, 121

Molecular cytogenetics, by FISH analysis, 133

Monocryl, 40

Monomorphic ventricular tachycardia, synchronized cardioversion and initial energy levels for, 33*t*

Monsel's solution, shave skin biopsy and, 51

Morphine, procedural sedation in adults and, 6*t*

Multiple sclerosis, diagnostic lumbar puncture and, 135

N

Nail elevator, ingrown toenails removal and, 65

Nail splitter, ingrown toenails removal and, 65

Nasostat catheter, 84

Neck extension, endotracheal intubation and, 11

Neurology procedures, 134–139
lumbar puncture, 135–139

Newborn circumcision, with Gomco clamp, 101–107

Noninvasive positive-pressure ventilation, 19–23
benefits, 19
BiPAP technique, *20*, 20–21, *21*
coding for, 23

complications of, minor and major, 22–23
contraindications, 19
CPAP technique, 22
definite indications (level 1 evidence), 19
equipment, 20
modes of, 20
monitoring patients on, 22
possible indications (level 2 evidence), 19
predictors of failure for, 22
references, 23
Nonpolyposis colon cancer syndrome, 114
NPPV. *See* Noninvasive positive-pressure ventilation

O

Obese patients, "ramp" position for intubation in, *14*
Obstructive lung disease, grading of spirometric abnormalities in, *168t*
Obstructive sleep apnea, endotracheal intubation and, 11
Obstructive ventilatory defect, spirograms, flow volume curves and, *167*
Onychocryptosis (ingrown toenails), 141
Opiates, moderate-deep sedation in adults and, 8
Opioids, mechanical ventilation and, 175
Orthopedics procedures, 140–163
arthrocentesis, 153–158
joint injections, 159–163
splinting and casting of extremities, 141–152
Otoscopy, 79

Oxygenation settings, mechanical ventilation, 175

P

PAC. *See* Pulmonary artery catheter
Pacing, transcutaneous, 35–37
Paddles, cardioversion and, in anterolateral position, *33*
Pancytopenia, unexplained, bone marrow aspiration/biopsy and, 127
Pap smear, 109–113
coding, 113
complications, 113
equipment, 109
indications, 109
liquid-based Pap testing, *112*
postprocedure evaluation, 113
preserving specimen, *112*
references, 113
relative contraindications, 109
sampling ectocervix with spatula, *110*
sampling endocervical canal with cytobrush, *110*
sampling endocervix and ectocervix with broom device, *111*
smearing sample on slide, *111*
traditional, technique, 109–112
Paracentesis, 87–93
ascitic fluid analysis, 91, *91t, 92t*
aspiration of ascitic fluid, *90*
coding, 92
complications
major, 91
minor, 92
contraindications, 87
diagnostic, indications, 87
equipment, 87

insertion sites, *88*
references, 93
technique, 88–89
therapeutic indications, 87
using evacuated container, *90*
when to use albumin, 89
Z tract method for insertion of paracentesis needle, *89*
Paragard T380A IUD
insertion
equipment, 118
preparing, *119*
technique, 119–120, *120*
replacement, 121
Paralytic agents, endotracheal intubation and, 17–18
PEEP-FiO$_2$ algorithm, for lung protective ventilation, *176t*
Pericardial fluid
analysis of, 30
aspiration of, *27*
Pericardiocentesis, 25–30
advancing dilator over wire, *28*
coding, 30
complications, 25
contraindications, 25
equipment, 26
indications, 25
pericardiocentesis catheter in place, *29*
pericardiocentesis catheter introduced over wire, *29*
references, 30
subxiphoid approach to, *27*
technique, 26
threading wire through the needle, *28*
Pericarditis
etiologies of, associated with large pericardial effusions, 25
work-up of, 30

Perivas fascia, stripping of, *98*

Phenol, nail ablation with, *67*

Pipelle, endometrial biopsy and, 114

Pipet Curet, endometrial biopsy and, 114

Plateau pressure, mechanical ventilation, 175

Pleural fluid
analysis of, 173
aspiration of, *172*
classification of, 173*t*

Pneumothorax
thoracentesis, and 173
tube thoracostomy and, 179

Polycythemia, unexplained, spirometry and, 165

Polymorphic ventricular tachycardia, synchronized cardioversion and initial energy levels for, 33*t*

Posterior epistaxis, 81
dual balloon nasal catheters and, *84*

Posterior leg and stirrup splints, *149, 150*

Posterior long arm splint, *148*

Posterior superior iliac spine, biopsy sites for, 128, *128*

Posterior superior iliac spine bone marrow aspirate, technique for, 129–130

Posterior superior iliac spine bone marrow biopsy, landmarks for, *128*

Posterior superior iliac spine bone marrow core biopsy technique, 130–133
advancing Jamshidi needle into bone marrow, *132*
advancing Jamshidi needle through bony cortex, *131*

pushing biopsy specimen out of Jamshidi needle, *132*
removing stylet from Jamshidi needle, *131*

PreservCyt solution, Pap smear and, 112

Pressure control (PC), mechanical ventilation, 175

Procedural sedation, 3–8
for abscesses, 70
airway assessment for potentially difficult oral intubation, 3, 5
anxiolysis in adults, 5
anxiolysis in children, 8
coding, 8
complications, 8
contraindications, 3
equipment, 5
indications, 3
levels of, 4*t*
medications for, in adults, 6*t*–7*t*
options for moderate-deep sedation in adults, 8
protocol, 5
references, 9

Prolene, 40

Propofol
endotracheal intubation and, 17
mechanical ventilation and, 175
moderate-deep sedation in adults and, 8
procedural sedation in adults and, 7*t*
synchronized cardioversion and, 32

Pseudotumor cerebri, diagnostic lumbar puncture and, 135

PSIS. *See* Posterior superior iliac spine

Pulmonary artery catheter
closing sterile sheath over, *207*
inserting through introducer sheath, *206*

insertion, 203–208
coding, 208
complications, 208
contraindications, absolute and relative, 203
equipment, 203–204
indications, 203
references, 208
technique, 204–208
natural curve at end of, *204*
placement of, best locations for, 205
sterile sheath placed over, *205*
waveforms configurations during insertion, *207*

Pulmonary artery catheter balloon, testing, *206*

Pulmonary procedures, 164–185
mechanical ventilation basics, 175–178
spirometry, 165–168
thoracentesis, 169–174
tube thoracostomy, 179–185

Punch skin biopsy, 59–62
anesthetizing skin, *60*
coding, 60
complications, 59
contraindications, 59
equipment, 59–60
indications, 59
performing punch biopsy, *61*
closing biopsy incision, *61*
excising skin biopsy, *61*
references, 62
technique, 60

Q

Q-tip application, cryosurgery and technique for, 47

R

Radial arterial line
advancing radial catheter over wire, *201*

arterial flash is seen, *199*
catheter insertion, *198*
connecting arterial
   catheter to pressure
   transducer tubing,
   201
technique for, *198–199*
wire threaded through
   arterial catheter
   and needle, *200*
wire threaded through
   arterial catheter
   needle, *200*
"Ramp" position, for
   intubation in
   morbidly obese
   patients, *14*
Ramsey Sedation scale, 176
Rapid-Pac, anterior
   epistaxis and, 82
Rapid Rhino, anterior
   epistaxis and, 82
Rapid sequence intubation,
   seven Ps of,
   12–14, 16
RASS. *See* Richmond
   Agitation-Sedation
   Scale
"Reflex" HPV DNA testing,
   Pap smear and,
   113
Restrictive lung disease,
   grading of
   spirometric
   abnormalities
   in, 167*t*
Restrictive ventilatory
   defect, spirograms,
   flow volume curves
   and, *167*
Rheumatoid arthritis,
   endotracheal
   intubation and, 11
Rhino Rocket, anterior
   epistaxis and, 82
Richmond Agitation-
   Sedation Scale, 176
Rise time, 21
Rocuronium, endotracheal
   intubation and, 13
"R on T" phenomenon,
   avoiding, 32
Rorcuronium, endotracheal
   intubation and, 18
Running stitch, *42*

S
SAAG. *See* Serum-ascites
   albumin gradient
SBT. *See* Spontaneous
   breathing trial
Scaphoid fractures,
   splinting for, 141
Seborrheic keratoses, 46
Sedation Agitation
   Scale, 176
Sedation levels, 4*t*
Seldinger technique,
   modified
brachial or femoral
   arterial line
   placement
   and, 200
central venous catheter
   placement and, 188
pulmonary artery catheter
   insertion and, 205
Sellick maneuver, 14
Serum-ascites albumin
   gradient, 91
Shave skin biopsy, 50–52
administering local
   anesthesia, *51*
coding, 52
complications, 52
contraindications, 50
equipment, 50
indications, 50
postprocedure care, 52
with razor blade, *51*
references, 52
with scalpel, *51*
technique, 50–51, *51*
Shock states, arterial line
   placement and, 197
Short arm cast, *148*
Short leg cast, *150*
Shoulder arthrocentesis
   technique for, 155–156
glenohumeral joint
   arthrocentesis-
   anterior approach,
   155
glenohumeral joint
   arthrocentesis-
   posterior approach,
   156
Simple interrupted suture,
   40, *41*
Simple running suture,
   40, *42*

Simplified Acute Physiology
   Score II (SAPSII),
   NPPV and, 22
SIMV. *See* Synchronized
   intermittent
   mandatory
   ventilation
Skin biopsies
excisional skin biopsy,
   53–58
punch skin biopsy, 59–62
shave skin biopsy, 50–52
Skin closure options, 40, *41,
   42, 43*
Skin lesions, cryosurgery of,
   46–49
Skin tags, 46
Sniffing position, for
   endotracheal
   intubation, 13, *13*
Sodium heparin (green-top)
   tube, bone marrow
   aspirate in, 133
Solar lentigo, 46
Spinal needle
insertion of, into L3-4
   interspace, *137*
manometer attached
   to, *137*
stylet removed from, *137*
Spirograms, flow volume
   curves and, *167*
Spirometer, use of, *166*
Spirometry, 165–168
acceptability criteria, 166
coding, 168
complications, 168
contraindications, 165
equipment, 165
indications, 165
interpretation of results,
   167
references, 168
reproducibility criteria,
   166
technique, 165–166
Splinting extremities
applying cast material
   for, *143*
basic technique for,
   142–144
coding, 151–152
complications, 151
contraindications, 141
equipment, 141

Splinting extremities—
    Continued
  indications, 141
  position of function of the
    hand, *142*
  postprocedure care, 151
  references, 152
  stockinette application,
    142
  wrap cast padding, *143*
  wrapping elastic wrap
    over cast material
    for, *144*
Spontaneous breathing trial,
  weaning/liberation
  from mechanical
  ventilators
  and, *177*
Squamous cell carcinomas,
  low-risk, shave skin
  biopsy and, 50
Sterilization, no-scalpel
  vasectomy and, 95
Sternal bone marrow
  sampling,
  contraindications,
  127
Sternum, biopsy sites
  for, 128
Stockinette
  applying, 142, *142*
  folding over cast
    material, *145*
  rolling cast material
    over, *146*
Stylet, endotracheal tube
  and, 15, 16
Subacromial bursa injection
  insertion site for, *161*
  lateral approach to, *161*
  technique, 160–161
Subacromial space,
  corticosteroids
  for, 160*t*
Subclavian vein catheters,
  193–194
  infraclavicular approach
    to, 193, *194*
  supraclavicular approach
    to, 193
Subcutaneous mass
  excision. *See*
  Lipoma or
  subcutaneous mass
  excision

Succinylcholine,
  endotracheal
  intubation and, 17
Sugar tong splint, *147*
Supraclavicular approach,
  to subclavian vein
  catheterization, 193
Supracondylar fractures,
  splinting for, 141
Supraventricular
  tachycardia,
  synchronized
  cardioversion and
  initial energy levels
  for, 33*t*
Surgilene, 40
Sutures
  chest tube secured
    with, *184*
  excisional skin biopsy
    and choice of, 54
  excision technique for
    large lipomas/
    subcutaneous
    masses and, 76
  horizontal mattress,
    40, *43*
  simple interrupted, 40, *41*
  simple running, 40, *42*
  size, choice of, 44
  timing removal of, 44
  vertical mattress, 40, *42*
Synchronized cardioversion,
  31–34
  coding, 34
  complications, 34
  contraindications
    to elective
    cardioversion, 31
  equipment, 31
  indications, 31
  placement of anterior-
    posterior pads
    for, *32*
  recommended initial
    energy levels
    for, 33*t*
  references, 34
  technique, 32–33
Synchronized intermittent
  mandatory
  ventilation, 175
Synovial fluid analysis,
  arthrocentesis
  and, 158

T
Talipes equinovarus, casting
  for, 141
Tenosynovitis, splinting
  for, 141
ThinPrep, Pap smear and,
  109
Thoracentesis, 169–174
  advancing needle into
    pleural space, *171*
  advancing thoracentesis
    catheter over
    needle, *171*
  aspiration of pleural
    fluid, *172*
  coding, 174
  complications, 173–174
  contraindications,
    absolute and
    relative, 169
  diagnostic, indications,
    169
  equipment, 169–170
  landmarks, *170*
  pleural fluid analysis/
    classification, 173,
    173*t*
  references, 174
  technique, 170–173
  therapeutic, *172*
    indications, 169
Thromboangiitis obliterans
  (Buerger disease),
  197
Thrombocytopenia,
  unexplained, bone
  marrow aspiration/
  biopsy and, 127
Thumb spica cast, *148*
Thyromental distance,
  endotracheal
  intubation and, 11
Tidal volume settings,
  mechanical
  ventilation, 175
Tissue adhesives, 40, *43*
TLC, restrictive lung disease
  and interpretation
  of, 167, 168*t*
Toenails, ingrown, removal
  of, 63–68
Transcutaneous pacing,
  35–37
  anterior-posterior pads
    placed for, *36*

anterolateral pads placed
for, *36*
coding, 37
complications, 37
contraindications, 35
equipment, 35
indications, 35
references, 37
rhythm strip
demonstrating good
pacing capture, *37*
rhythm strip with pacing
spikes and no
capture, *37*
technique, 35–36, *36*
Transudates, causes of, 173
Trephines
sizes, for punch skin
biopsies, 59
technique, for punch skin
biopsies, 60
Triggering sensitivity, 21
Trochanteric bursa injection
insertion site, *162*
technique, 163
Tube thoracostomy,
179–185
blunt dissection during
chest tube
placement, *183*
chest tube insertion, *183*
chest tube placement,
proper position
for, *181*
chest tube
troubleshooting,
182
coding, 185
complications, major and
minor, 185
contraindications, 179
discontinuation of chest
tubes, 184–185
equipment, 179–180
indications, 179
local anesthesia for chest
tube placement,
181
references, 185

securing chest tube
suture, *184*
skin incision for chest
tube placement,
182
technique, 180–182
Tympanograms, types of, *80*
Tympanometer with
printer, 79
Tympanometry, 79–80
coding, 79
complications, 79
contraindications, 79
equipment, 79
indications, 79
references, 80
technique, 79

U

Ulnar gutter splint, *147*

V

Vaginal bleeding, abnormal,
evaluation of, 114
Vascular procedures,
186–196
arterial line placement,
197–202
central venous access,
187–196
intraosseous line
placement,
209–212
pulmonary artery catheter
insertion, 203–208
Vas deferens
cauterizing ends of, *99*
excising segment of, *99*
isolated, ligating, *99*
three-finger grasp of, *96*
Vasectomy, no-scalpel,
95–100
anesthesia of vas, *97*
cauterizing ends of
vas, *99*
coding, 100
complications, 100
contraindications, 95
equipment, 95

excising segment of the
vas, *99*
grasping vas, *98*
holding vas, *96*
indications, 95
ligating isolated vas, *99*
postprocedure care, 100
references, 100
stripping of perivas
fascia, *98*
technique, 95–99
Vasectomy clamp, vas
grasped with, *98*
VDRL, CSF studies and, 138
Vecuronium, endotracheal
intubation and, 13
Ventilator rate setting, 175
Vertical mattress suture,
40, *42*
Vertigo, tympanometry and
evaluation of, 79
Vicryl, 40
Vicryl sutures, excision
technique for
large lipomas/
subcutaneous
masses and, 76
Video laryngoscopy, 11
Volar short arm splint, *147*

W

Webril
applying, 143, *143*
cast material applied
over, *145*
folding over cast
material, *145*
rolling cast material
over, *146*
"Wineglass position,"
splinting and,
142, *142*
Wrap cast padding (Webril),
143, *143*

Z

Z tract method, inserting
paracentesis needle
and, 88, *89*

Stay Connected with Tarascon Publishing!

Monthly Dose eNewsletter
—Tarascon's Monthly eNewsletter

Stay up-to-date and subscribe today at: <u>www.tarascon.com</u>

Written specifically with Tarascon customers in mind, the Tarascon Monthly Dose will provide you with new drug information, tips and tricks, updates on our print, mobile and online products as well as some extra topics that are interesting and entertaining.

Sign up to receive the Tarascon Monthly Dose Today! Simply register at <u>www.tarascon.com</u>.

You can also stay up-to-date with Tarascon news, new product releases, and relevant medical news and information on Facebook, Twitter page, and our Blog.

STAY CONNECTED

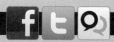

Facebook: www.facebook.com/tarascon
Twitter: @JBL_Medicine
Blog: portfolio.jblearning.com/medicine